Eldercare, Health, and Ecosyndemics in a Perilous World

Environmental Health in a Changing World

Series Editor: Merrill Singer

Senior Research Scientist, Center for Health, Intervention and Prevention; Professor, Departments of Anthropology and Community Health, University of Connecticut

The Environmental Health in a Changing World series consists of volumes that address significant and emergent issues in environmental health as seen through the anthropological lens and as responded to through the application of anthropology to helping solve environmental health problems in diverse populations. Environmental health has become a key concept for understanding health in the modern world as a result of the role of human activities in producing adverse changes in the environment. The negative health consequences of environmental factors—or more specifically, anthropogenic environmental factors—are growing at an ever-increasing pace due to climate change. Climatic change of the magnitude projected by climate scientists, for example, will have severe consequences for human well-being around the world. In this light, anthropologists have been playing an expanding role in understanding and addressing environmental health challenges around the globe and with reference to a wide range of environmental health issues. The anthropological approach that unites the books in this series begins with a recognized need to learn the perspective of impacted populations. How do they view local and global environments, environmental health risks, and effective responses? As a result of this concern, the anthropological perspective draws attention to what health statistics alone cannot tell us. It does this by ensuring that people—as experiencing, feeling, and self-aware beings—are not lost in the epidemiological and public health analysis of morbidity and mortality data.

Eldercare, Health, and Ecosyndemics in a Perilous World

Janelle Christensen

ROWMAN & LITTLEFIELD
Lanham • Boulder • New York • London

Published by Rowman & Littlefield
An imprint of The Rowman & Littlefield Publishing Group, Inc.
4501 Forbes Boulevard, Suite 200, Lanham, Maryland 20706
www.rowman.com

Unit A, Whitacre Mews, 26-34 Stannary Street, London SE11 4AB, United Kingdom

British Library Cataloguing in Publication Information Available

Library of Congress Cataloging-in-Publication Data

Names: Christensen, Janelle, 1979– author.
Title: Eldercare, health, and ecosyndemics in a perilous world / Janelle Christensen.
Description: Lanham : Rowman & Littlefield, [2018] | Series: Environmental health in a changing world | Includes bibliographical references and index.
Identifiers: LCCN 2018023052 (print) | LCCN 2018031500 (ebook) | ISBN 9780759123946 (electronic) | ISBN 9780759123939 (cloth) | ISBN 9781538158487 (pbk)
Subjects: LCSH: Environmental health. | Older people—Effect of environment on. | Older people—Care. | Aging.
Classification: LCC RA566 (ebook) | LCC RA566 .C568 2018 (print) | DDC 613/.0438—dc23
LC record available at https://lccn.loc.gov/2018023052

Contents

Preface

My most recent research, conducted between 2009 and 2011, was specifically on how people with Alzheimer's disease and their informal (often family) caregivers prepared for hurricanes in Southeast Florida. Though not included in my research, my own great uncle was living in an independent living facility outside Miami with my great aunt. He had Parkinson's disease, which caused an associated dementia. My husband's grandmother was diagnosed with vascular dementia and was moved out of her home in the Midwest and into his parents' home in Florida. None of those who participated in my research (or my own family members) experienced a hurricane (or other weather-related disaster) during this time. My great aunt and uncle moved to a state up north to be closer to their adult children. My husband's grandmother passed on. Her younger cousin, also living in Florida, was diagnosed with Alzheimer's disease shortly thereafter. In all these cases, difficult, stressful decisions were made to provide the best care possible. Providing care within the context of climate change, with sharper and more prolonged temperature extremes, will make survival and quality of life more difficult, especially for our elders.

Research takes place within the context of the researchers' lived lives. This is especially salient when doing research with living populations (as opposed to studying the past). My research with people with disabilities, caregivers, and others living with a long-term illness is interwoven with my personal life. After experiencing Hurricane Irma in 2017 with my children, watching my neighbors and extended family contend with the difficult decision to evacuate or remain at home, it was powerfully clear how much more difficult age-related illnesses and disabilities become during a crisis.

The connections I make within this book are informed both by my own structured research, the work of other academic researchers, the stories filtered through the lens of journalism, and my own personal experiences in my community before, during, and after Hurricane Irma in 2017, a storm that paled in comparison to Hurricane Maria, which followed.

CHRISTENSEN FIELD NOTES, SEPTEMBER 6, 2017

Hurricane Irma is projected to hit south Florida on 9-9-17. As my family prepares for a potential hit, the theme of Gregory Button's "Disaster Culture" returns to mind: uncertainty (Button 2010). It is difficult to make decisions with incomplete information. Often, we fill in the gaps with hopeful thinking, or, other times, with fear of the worst. Even after studying how people prepare and respond to disasters for almost a decade, I find myself having very little voice within my own family: they have experienced hurricanes, and I have not. Though each storm is unique and the biggest mistakes are usually made making decisions based on positive past experiences, I find myself standing with my family rather than the gut instinct that is born of years of studying empirical research (Eisenman et al. 2007; Dash and Gladwin 2007; Christensen, Richey, and Castaneda 2013). I understand now, more than I ever had, how people find themselves placed in danger's way, making decisions within their family unit.

Hurricane Irma caused considerable conflict in my family. The models changed daily, sometimes suggesting it would hit West Palm Beach or, possibly, Miami. Then, it shifted, threatening to bisect the state of Florida. While my family was relieved by this model, I was not; I knew the threat posed to the area by Lake Okeechobee, a shallow but very large body of water in the center of Florida. The 1928 hurricane hit the lake directly, causing mass destruction in the surrounding areas (Mykle 2002; Kleinberg 2003). Though the Army Corps of Engineers had been draining the lake in anticipation of hurricane season and a stronger dike had been under construction for years, Irma's current track did not ease my mind ("U.S. Army Corps of Engineers Jacksonville District" 2010, "Herbert Hoover Dike Major Rehabilitation Evaluation Report" 2000; Stapleton 2017). I knew that this area was second only to New Orleans in vulnerability to a hurricane (Zhang, Xiao, and Leatherman 2006; Leatherman, Zhang, and Xiao 2007). My husband admonished me to find a history of flooding resulting from Lake Okeechobee affecting the Gulf Coast side of the state. I pointed out that flood maps everywhere had to be rewritten after each hurricane, including Hurricane Katrina and Hurricane Sandy (Jonkman et al. 2009; Cobb 2013). The news was still covered with the catastrophic images of a flooded Houston, Texas, brought on by Hurricane Harvey (McCausland and Chuck 2017; McGraw and Ghebremedhin 2017). My in-laws, a healthy, active couple in their sixties, did not plan to leave their home (my mother-in-law was particularly annoyed that her triathlon was canceled because of Hurricane Irma). They had successfully weathered Hurricane Charley over a decade before and felt confident they had what they needed in place to shelter at their home.

Even as the model shifted, indicating that Hurricane Irma would make a direct hit in either Fort Myers or Naples, Florida, where we lived, they insisted on sheltering in place. Storm surge predictions began to headline the newspaper (Fountain 2017). On Friday, August 8, there was a mandatory evacuation order for my neighborhood, but my in-laws' area, a mile away, remained in a separate zone and was not ordered to evacuate.

My husband, assessing the mandatory evacuation order and the predicted storm surge (and perhaps reacting to my passive-aggressive question "why did I bother spending a decade in graduate school studying this if I can't get my own children to safety?"), agreed to evacuate. We left that morning for the inland city of Orlando (north of Lake Okeechobee). We called hotel chains from our cell phones while on the road and secured a room. The roads were clear (enough that I took photos to send to family members who claimed they could not evacuate because of the congested roads—it did not convince them to evacuate). From the road, I was texted by cousins in Georgia and the Carolinas about their parents who, like my in-laws, were refusing to leave their coastal homes in Florida, despite their adult children's pleas. By late afternoon, my in-laws had also received an evacuation order. A neighbor later told me that a police car drove slowly through the neighborhoods, encouraging people to leave by loudspeakers. My in-laws joined us by nightfall, where we sheltered in the hotel. On Sunday, my children slept through the storm, hardly bothered by the rattling of the windows.

Even with our excellent warning systems, assessing our risk and agreeing on a response to an impending hurricane was wrought with conflict. With an increased population and sprawling development, the potential for a difficult evacuation and extensive damage was great. My area was fortunate in a way that the city of Houston or the entire territory of Puerto Rico was not. Houston was inundated with floods. At the time of writing (February 2018), Puerto Rico remains without power. In May 2018, a Harvard study reported the death toll there was close to 4,645 people (Kishore et al. 2018). The report indicated most of them were elders, succumbing to the heat and lack of available medical services.

THE GLOBAL AND THE PERSONAL

Since I began writing this book in 2013, a lot has changed for me personally, in the measures of climate change, and in the political environment. When I began writing in 2013, I wrote about how the warmest year on record was in 2010 ("Global Climate Report—Annual 2013" 2014). By the end of 2013, the 2010 record was broken (Cole and McCarthy 2014). The following year, 2014, I saw the birth of my first child and, also, the warmest year since 1880 (Cole and McCarthy 2015). In 2015, I had my second child and, as the year ended, the record for the warmest year had been shattered (Brown, Cabbage, and McCarthy 2016). When my family and I relocated to another setting in 2016, the average global temperature rose *again* (Potter, Cabbage, and McCarthy 2017). According to the January 18, 2017, NASA news conference, "the planet's average surface temperature has risen about 2.0 degrees Fahrenheit (1.1 degrees Celsius) since the late 19th century" (Potter, Cabbage, and McCarthy 2017, para. 6). Shortly before submitting a draft of this book to my editors in 2017, we watched as Hurricane Harvey flooded Houston. A week later, we evacuated our Florida home as Hurricane Irma was set to make landfall on the west coast of the state.

Despite the upward global temperature trend, climate science remains in a politically tenuous position, with climate scientists themselves sometimes threatened with frivolous lawsuits and death threats (Kurtz 2016; Milman 2017; Clynes 2012). Powerful fossil fuel lobbies, such as Koch Industries, Peabody Coal, Arch Coal, and Alpha Natural Resources, have used multi-pronged attacks to sow confusion about climate science in the United States and abroad (covered in chapter 4) (Monbiot 2006, 2009; Oreskes and Conway 2010a). In 2017, evidence was released showing ExxonMobil knew burning fossil fuels (releasing CO_2 into the atmosphere) could contribute to a warmer climate but hid that information (Supran and Oreskes 2017).

In November 2015, the Canadian government shifted from the conservative leadership of Stephen Harper to the liberal leadership of Justin Trudeau (Jones 2016). Harper, much like the United States' 43rd president, George W. Bush, had placed restrictions on climate researchers speaking to the public about climate change. Trudeau withdrew those restrictions, just as the Obama administration had in the United States in 2008 when Barack Obama first took office. One of Trudeau's first actions as prime minister of Canada was to attend the Paris Climate Conference (also called Conference of the Parties or COP21) ("United Nations Climate Change Conference Paris 2015" 2015).

In December 2015, signatories of the Paris Accord, an agreement between 196 representative governments in the United Nations, agreed to the goal of reducing greenhouse emissions and preventing a rise of two degrees Celsius average temperature (UNFCC 2015). The agreement strengthened support to developing nations, such as India, to increase their clean energy sources (e.g., solar power plants). On November 4, 2016, the Paris Accord entered into force, indicating that at least fifty-five countries accounting for at least 55 percent of the total global greenhouse emissions had ratified the agreement ("Paris Agreement—Status of Ratification" 2016).

A new prime minister, Malcom Turnbull, was sworn into office in Australia in September 2015 (BBC News 2015). Though previously a proponent of climate science, the *Guardian*'s Graham Readfearn noted a shift in Turnbull's stance, when Turnbull adopted pro-coal narratives (2017). Indeed, his stance would become even more pro–oil production in 2017 (Williams 2017). However, his energy minister, Josh Frydenberg, said that Australia remained committed to the Paris Accord in 2017 (Chan 2017).

In June 2016, Great Britain voted to leave the European Union, a move commonly referred to as Brexit. The effect of Brexit on environmental regulations remain in question because "membership of the EU has had a fundamental impact on environmental legislation in the UK. . . . UK climate change policy has also become increasingly enmeshed in EU policy" (House of Lords 2017). Reports, however, suggest that climate change regulations are to be "scaled down" once Brexit goes into effect (Revesz 2017).

The Obama administration, which had prioritized climate change as a policy issue, gave way to the vehemently antienvironmental-regulation Trump administration. Environmental scientists and college students frantically began to back up the accumulated climate data collected during the Obama administration, fearing the Trump administration would destroy it (Dennis 2016). Further stoking fears, in March 2017, President Donald Trump struck down six measures that Obama had put in place to protect the environments surrounding coal mines (BBC News 2017). Trump appointed Scott Pruitt, a skeptic of climate change, to lead the Environmental Protection Agency (EPA) (Davenport and Lipton 2016). He also appointed an ExxonMobil executive, Rex Tillerson, as Secretary of State. Despite his fossil fuel background, Tillerson made public statements supporting the validity of climate change and encouraged the president to remain in the Paris Accord (Tollefson 2017).

After Trump's win in the United States, several far-right candidates, primarily running on anti-immigrant and antirefugee platforms, appeared to gain some traction in Europe: Geert Wilders in the Netherlands and Marine Le Pen in France (Connolly 2017). Though not central to the platform, right-wing populism threatened the Paris Climate Agreement in Europe as well (Light 2017). Both shared a distrust of multinational agreements or bodies such as the United Nations, European Union, and Paris Accord. In March 2017, Wilders failed to defeat Mark Rutte's "center right" VVD party (Chappell 2017). Two months later, independent centrist Emmanuel Macron defeated the far-right, nationalist candidate, Le Pen, for the French presidential election (Chrisafis 2017).

The world watched closely as the newly elected world leaders gathered in Brussels for the NATO summit in May 2017 ("Meeting of Heads of State and/or Government" 2017). By June 2017, Trump announced that he would withdraw the United States from the Paris Climate Agreement (Shear 2017). By most assessments, Trump cannot make a unilateral withdrawal from the Paris Accord, and "it does not signal the unraveling of the global climate change governance system" (Betsill 2017, 189). The symbolic and diplomatic standing of the United States internationally, however, does not appear to be as resilient.

In August 2017 the sequel to Al Gore's *Inconvenient Truth, An Inconvenient Sequel,* hit theaters. The film documents some of the events I mention above (the Paris Accord, in particular) and incorporates several climate-related events that I write about in the following chapters. This book is different in that its focus is on the work of archaeologists, anthropologists, and other researchers, demonstrating the impact of climate change on the earth's most vulnerable populations. Climate change is not something far off that could happen; anthropologists see how it impacts people they work with and care about *now.* Anthropologists write about the Sakha of Northeastern Siberia, Russia, where grazing fields for animals are "increasingly inundated with water," to the San of the Kalahari Desert, who like many on the African continent depend on immediately available natural resources (Crate 2009; Hitchock 2009).

I also worked with people affected by a disrupted climate, though closer to home: elders who live along the Florida coast. Nearly every month, more scientific evidence becomes available, outlining how sea level rise impacts the state in which I live (Wdowinski et al. 2016). A recent study explored why sea level rise is higher in the Miami area than in some other coastal areas and that "significant changes in flooding frequency occurred after 2006" (Valle-Levinson, Dutton, and Martin 2017). The current governor of this state, Rick Scott, and one of its senators, Marco Rubio, both express doubt about the reality of climate change, even as the streets of Miami now regularly flood (Mooney and Rein 2017). I wonder if it is safe for my older family members to remain here. Given the widespread disruption in the climate and the many ways in which climate-related events can endanger older populations, where is it safer to grow old? If there is no clear answer to this question, we need to address why there is resistance to curbing the underlying causes of climate change.

It was in this context, one in which we understand the human vulnerability to extreme weather events—one in which we know extreme weather events will become more frequent—that close to five thousand American citizens died in Puerto Rico (Kishore et al. 2018). Most of these deaths were preventable and were due to lack of services.

SUMMARY

Anthropology is uniquely situated to explore how the changing climate affects societies because it is holistic; it draws upon and informs not only the explanatory stories that give humans meaning but also the biology, ecology, psychology, sociology, economics, engineering, chemistry, mythology, and sociolegal structures, as well as political-economic and historical contexts. It connects how the human body works biologically and socially within the context of its environment. Anthropologists provide insights to environments of the past, how previous societies responded to those environments, and compares those trends to the present. We also compare across existing cultures to shine light on our own societies' strengths and potential deficiencies, including the mobilization of social hierarchies, economic systems, gender roles, and life course issues that either reduce or amplify morbidity and mortality. We share how other societies respond to environmental pressures in the past through archaeology. Yet there has been an obfuscation of the science as it is communicated to some sectors of the population.

A theoretical orientation toward critical medical anthropology means understanding dementia within a social and historical context. Over the course of my dissertation research and beyond, it became clear that Alzheimer's disease was not the only chronic illness that affected older individuals during extreme weather events. Even the gradual loss of eyesight, part of the normal aging process, can pose a challenge during extreme weather events. A chronic, long-term, progressive disease makes evacuation particularly difficult and dangerous. Furthermore, hurricanes are not the only threat people face in a changing climate. My research fit within an overarching pattern of heightened vulnerability at a time when extreme weather events, including heat waves, blizzards, flooding, and droughts, are becoming more frequent and, potentially, more extreme.

As populations age, not just in the United States but internationally, it is important to understand the unique risks these populations face. The combination of dense, largely older populations in coastal urban centers during a time of global climate change presents an opportunity for a perfect storm of vulnerable situations to form. This perfect storm contains all the elements necessary to be categorized as an ecosyndemic (Singer 2008; Singer 2010; Baer and Singer 2014). An ecosyndemic is a way of explaining how a physical body exists within its social and ecological conditions and how those conditions can amplify a disease process. It incorporates the concept of ecology and syndemics, which is when two coexisting diseases interact in a symbiotic manner to ultimately amplify morbidity, mortality, and human suffering overall (see chapter 2) (Singer et al. 2006; Singer 2009).

As the climate is disrupted, stronger storms and unusual weather conditions are increasingly striking vulnerable areas. This is exacerbated by rising sea levels. Hurricanes (and post-hurricane conditions) can, in turn, exacerbate underlying age-related illnesses, such as heart disease. As there are now larger populations of elderly individuals living in vulnerable areas, emergency managers need to be aware of how environmental changes can amplify the impact of disease, creating clusters of suffering.

As will be discussed in chapter 7, researchers and lawmakers must take care that the concept of vulnerability does not become a "cause of death." Rather, it should be used as a tool to identify and mitigate underlying problems. Lakshmi Fjord's concept of the "expected dead," where excess deaths among the elderly and disabled are shrugged off as the natural order of things, is central. Vulnerability, such as an upper respiratory illness, is usually temporary; if the illness strikes during an inopportune time, such as after a hurricane, the result can be deadly. Fjord and Manderson (2009) suggest that researchers and first responders reframe the concept of vulnerability to "vulnerable situations" rather than "vulnerable people" (a concept first deployed by Wisner et al. 2004).

Chapter One

Betsy and Joe, and the Elder Health Ecosyndemic

As I was embarking on my dissertation research, in partnership with an organization called Alzheimer's Community Care, I was invited to join a group of caregivers traveling to Tallahassee, Florida. On this trip, I met "Betsy." In March 2011, I walked into a Florida state representative's office in Tallahassee with Betsy, her photographs, and the supervisor of the adult day care center, Ron Radcliffe. We explained the importance of the Silver Alert Bill, which would provide law enforcement with resources to aid in locating and returning missing elders. Our secondary goal was to lobby for the continuation of funding for adult day care programs and caregiver support. Funding for these programs had been cut every year since 2007, totaling in a 42 percent cut in state funding (Radcliffe 2011). The representative listened politely, and then asked, "Shouldn't we be prioritizing funding to find a cure for Alzheimer's, not just on maintaining the status quo?" I made a clumsy attempt at explaining the difference between "healing" (treating the person) and "curing" (treating the disease) but I stopped myself; my argument was a critique of biomedicine, which often fails to address the actual suffering of individuals as it pursues a cure (Kleinman 1980).

Anthropologists distinguish between disease (the objective, biological symptoms) and illness (the socially defined significance and response to the disease) (Kleinman 1980). To put it another way, "medical anthropologists do not dispute that biological disease occurs but are more interested in the reasons why scientifically demonstrable physical pathology should appear and be treated in such different ways around the world" (Hashmi 2009, 207).

However, I only had five minutes of face time with the representative, and I quickly realized I had been operating under one set of assumptions about the disease and he, another. To ask someone to, in five minutes, reflect upon and critique the assumptions he has carried for approximately fifty years was simply too much. It was beyond the scope of our meeting to address disparate worldviews. Instead, we argued that, until there is a cure, spending money to support family caregivers would cost less than formal institutionalization of people with Alzheimer's disease or a related dementia (Radcliffe 2011). This state senator did, ultimately, vote in favor of our proposed legislation. Many did, regardless of party. During our short meetings with them two other state senators revealed they also had a parent diagnosed with Alzheimer's disease.

Though I did not have time to explain the nuances of disease and illness in our meetings, in the following pages I will take the time to discuss the historical framing of "old age" and age-related diseases that I could not with the senator. This includes (but is not limited to) Alzheimer's disease (and related dementias). I will explain the (medical) anthropological underpinnings of concepts like "old" and "senile," "sick" and "well" (Kleinman 1980). The concept of a "social construction" does not mean that "aging" or "Alzheimer's disease" are "not real," but rather that their content depends upon historical and social contingencies that may shift over time, location, and cultural context (Kleinman 1980). Because of these socially contingent definitions, we make assumptions about what illnesses are and *how people with these conditions ought to be treated*. This also has implications for *applied solutions*, since a problem based on a set of social assumptions often requires *a shift in perspective* and definitions to resolve conflict. These concepts from classical medical anthropology will be filtered through the specific theoretical lens of critical medical anthropology. I then lead into the historical construction of aging, health, and illness, using Alzheimer's type dementia as a primary example. I specifically consider the idea of "normal aging" and how it is juxtaposed against "age-related diseases."

"Betsy and Joe Dunmore's" story can provide insight into these perspectives. Betsy (not her real name) agreed to two interviews with me for my dissertation research and completed a survey (described in Christensen 2012). Many of the details of their lives have been changed to protect their identities, but their core experiences as a couple dealing with a progressive, chronic disease in a changing climate are true.

Betsy and Joe Dunmore had lived a successful and full life in Montana. The Dunmores, however, had had their fill of the cold and decided to relocate to sunnier shores. They settled on a lovely home in a gated community along part of the 8,436 miles of coastal shoreline that is Florida ("Ocean and Coastal Management in Florida" 2012). Shortly before they moved in 2003, Joe was officially diagnosed with Alzheimer's type dementia, which would eventually render him unable to care for himself. They decided to move south despite Joe's life-altering diagnosis. According to the state's website, about one thousand people move to Florida each day, presumably to chase the sun ("Facts About Florida," n.d.). Some migrate from the surrounding Caribbean islands in search of more lucrative jobs.

Geographers have watched the increasing number of people living near the coast with concern, noting that these areas are inherently vulnerable to hurricanes, floods, and other disasters (Uitto 1998; Wisner and Uitto 2009). Indeed, the four most populous states, California, Texas, New York, and Florida, are coastal and contain what are considered "megacities," such as Los Angeles and Miami (Uitto and Shaw 2006).

The vulnerability of coastal megacities was not a prominent concern when Joe and Betsy decided to make their move. They were focused on relocating, Joe's diagnosis, and estate planning.

As the Dunmores settled into their new home near Florida's east coast, they found new routines. They went to the community center on Thursdays for dinner with other community members. As the months wore on, Joe became more forgetful and eventually began to bow out of their routine dinners. Though he still enjoyed his morning walks, he did little more than wave at the neighbors. Once an active and social man, most of his time was now spent staring out the window or watching television.

One morning, Joe went on his morning walk and did not return. After he had been gone for over an hour, Betsy began searching for him, first on foot, knocking on neighbors' doors, then, with increasing alarm, by car. The guard who greeted incoming cars at the community gate said she had seen Joe walk out toward the road. Betsy located her disoriented husband over two miles from their home. After that incident, Betsy went with him on his walks. Later, she learned that 60 percent of people with Alzheimer's disease will wander at some point during the disease (Aud 2004; Rowe et al. 2011; McShane et al. 1998).

In the summer of 2004, Betsy watched the news with increasing concern; the reports indicated that Hurricane Charley was predicted to hit Florida. Since the Dunmores had never experienced a hurricane, Betsy listened attentively to the preparation instructions. Though the projected path did not appear to directly threaten their home, Betsy was concerned and began searching for the protective hurricane panels that had come with her home. Betsy found the large, heavy panels in the garage, along with an instructional videotape. Betsy was frustrated when she realized she was unable to lift the panels on her own and Joe was unable to assist her. She knocked on her neighbor's door, the home of a single woman in her sixties. Together, Betsy and her neighbor watched an instructional video on how to install the panels over the large windows. They struggled to lift and secure the unwieldy panels over the vulnerable glass windows and sliding doors. It took them two days to install all of them. The result was a very dark home without natural light; however, the windows would be protected from any flying objects dislodged in high winds associated with hurricanes. Joe seemed agitated by the change, repeatedly asking questions about the dark.

When Betsy went to her neighbor's home to return the favor, they found that it didn't have hurricane panels. The neighboring home had been built a year before the Dunmores', and the building codes in their county had not yet required hurricane panels, hurricane shutters, or impact-resistant glass in home construction. Florida building codes were updated in 1992, after Hurricane Andrew (Tsikoudakis 2012).

Though they were under a hurricane watch for a few days, Hurricane Charley was not expected to make a direct hit in their area. On August 13, 2004, Betsy, Joe, and their neighbor watched the news in horror as Hurricane Charley crashed into the coast opposite their homes. They were not ordered to evacuate, so they stayed in their homes. The images of the devastation and downed buildings kept them rapt as they flipped through the channels. When it was clear they were no longer in danger, Betsy and her neighbor struggled to remove the heavy hurricane panels.

Less than three weeks later, a second hurricane, Frances, formed in the Atlantic. This time, the Dunmores' home was in the hurricane's projected direct path, in the center of the "cone of uncertainty" that flashed across their television screens. Again, Betsy and her neighbor danced with the hurricane panels. As the storm approached the news went from a hurricane watch to a hurricane warning. According to NOAA, a hurricane watch means that hurricane conditions are *possible* within 48 hours; when a hurricane warning is issued, a hurricane is *expected within 36* hours and preparations are advised. A mandatory evacuation order was issued, and Betsy started packing the car. Joe watched in growing consternation as she loaded supplies and shuffled around the home.

"I'm not going anywhere," Joe told his wife.

"But we have to. The storm is coming right at us! Look at the news!"

They argued for over an hour, Joe refusing to leave his chair or his home. Betsy was beside herself. Joe was a large man. There was no way she could force him, even if she had wanted to. She went to the bedroom to collect her thoughts and calm herself after an exhausting argument.

After some time, she casually went into the living room and switched the television to an old movie. She went to the kitchen and made some lunch.

"Joe, how about we go get some ice cream? We don't even have to get out of the car. We can go through the drive-through."

Joe agreed and accompanied her to the packed and loaded car. In search of ice cream, Betsy drove by the fast-food restaurants where she normally would buy it, but they were closed while the area was under a hurricane warning. She was forced to drive on to the emergency shelter, run by the American Red Cross. She brought Joe to the registration desk, where two young children screamed as they pulled at each other's shirts. The large area had high ceilings and the sound carried throughout the converted school gym. Uncertainly, Betsy fumbled with registration forms with the help of a volunteer. She could see all of the mats laid out on the floor. Joe looked completely flustered and disoriented in the noise and chaos.

"I'm sorry," Betsy said to the volunteer. "I can't do this. I can't make Joe sleep on the floor. He has a hard time getting out of a regular bed . . . and the noise . . ."

"Where will you go?" the volunteer asked.

"I don't know."

Unfortunately, the American Red Cross volunteer could not offer any solutions because this county did not have a special needs shelter that could accommodate Joe or anyone else with Alzheimer's type dementia. Even if it had, it is possible that the volunteer might not have been aware of it because in Florida special needs shelters are run through county emergency operations centers, not directly through the American Red Cross like regular shelters.

Betsy returned home and called her daughter in Montana. Together, they began calling different hotels across Florida. Her daughter was able to secure a room across the state. Betsy was deeply thankful for their healthy bank account that would allow them to pay for safe, secure, private, and quiet shelter.

In their attempt to cross the state to a safer location, the Dunmores discovered they were not the only family with this plan; they encountered gridlock traffic. Joe was upset, deeply confused, and uncomfortable. There were approximately 2.5 million people ordered to evacuate Florida's southeast coast (Moser 2004). Betsy was near tears between the frustration of negotiating the road with so many other cars, Joe's incessant questions, and her flustered responses. What was normally a two-hour drive had become a strenuous eight-hour journey. When they eventually made it to the hotel room, Joe went straight to the bed and lay down facing the wall. Other than going to the bathroom, which he had trouble finding, he refused to move. When he did try to find the bathroom, he sometimes mistook the exit door as the bathroom door. Betsy, terrified that Joe would accidentally leave the hotel room thinking it was the bathroom, remained ever vigilant. She slept very little during their stay at the hotel.

Hurricane Frances hit Florida on the border of Martin and St. Lucie counties on September 5, 2004 (Barnes 2007). When it made landfall, it was listed as a category 2 storm on the Saffir-Simpson scale. However, it was a "wet" storm, with torrential rain and storm surges. Florida Power and Light reported power outages to 659,000 customers in Palm Beach, 590,000 in Broward, 423,000 in Miami-Dade, 39,200 in Collier, 2,500 in Hendry, and 1,700 in Glades counties. An estimated 17,000 persons sought refuge in public shelters in Palm Beach County and nearly 7,000 in Broward County (Beven 2004). Ultimately, Hurricane Frances caused an estimated $12 billion (2004 USD) in damage (Barnes 2007).

When the Dunmores returned to their home, they found it secure. They had lost the screen that protected their porch and pool area, but the panels had protected their windows from flying objects or any potential looters. The mangroves that lined the coast in this area had helped to disperse the storm surge that otherwise would have flooded their home.

Regardless, they were without power for nearly a week after they returned. Without power, they were without air-conditioning. Betsy struggled to keep Joe hydrated in the sweltering, humid Florida summer heat, constantly handing him cups of water. Fortunately, the frequent rainstorms helped to keep the overall temperatures from becoming heat waves, which could pose a serious threat to health, especially for older populations.

Joe asked for his radio, for music, for television, none of which were available without electricity, and he could not remember why they were not available. Luckily, he never got sick of the peanut butter and jelly sandwiches that served as both lunch and dinner, every day while the power remained out. Betsy, however, had difficulty enjoying them after the 2004 hurricane season.

Two weeks later, Hurricane Ivan hit the Florida Panhandle on the Alabama border on September 16, 2004. Though Ivan had fluctuated between category 3 and 5 during its life, it was a category 3 on the Saffir-Simpson scale when it hit (Stewart 2005). In total, Hurricane Ivan was directly responsible for ninety-one deaths in the Caribbean and twenty-five deaths in the United States. Most of the US deaths were due to the tornadoes associated with the hurricane (McKinney, Houser, and Meyer-Arendt 2011). The Dunmores were unaffected by Hurricane Ivan; however, they nervously watched the news. Betsy was too exhausted to be shocked when news came of a fourth hurricane, Jeanne, which was forecast to hit them as directly as Hurricane Frances had a few weeks before.

Betsy found herself, once again, struggling with the hurricane panels. She debated whether she should evacuate Joe again, even though there were mandatory evacuation orders for their area. Her blood pressure had been elevated over the past few months and she was physically, mentally, and emotionally exhausted. Her role as a caregiver was exhausting enough. Caring for someone with Alzheimer's disease or a related dementia often results in exacerbating health conditions of the caregiver. This type of caregiving has some of the highest caregiver burden measured (Etters, Goodall, and Harrison 2008). Adding the stress of multiple hurricanes was almost unbearable. Joe would not be any more enthusiastic about leaving the familiar surroundings of home where, if nothing else, he could usually locate the bathroom. Betsy discussed the decision with her daughter; after all, Betsy argued, the house had withstood the impact of Hurricane Frances . . . she wanted to believe that they would be safe in a familiar environment. Over the phone, her daughter begged her to heed the official evacuation orders. Betsy was not the only person who was reluctant to evacuate again. Studies have shown that individuals who have weathered previous hurricanes tend to be less likely to evacuate in the future (Dash and Gladwin 2007). Some have called this trend "hurricane amnesia" or "risk fatigue" (Christensen 2012).

Betsy watched through the window as her neighbor packed her car. Reluctantly, she did the same. This time, she was careful to pack bags out of Joe's sight so that he would not become agitated. Her daughter, once again, assisted her with finding a hotel room on the other side of the state.

On September 25, 2004, Jeanne hit Florida as a category 3 hurricane on the Saffir-Simpson scale (Barnes 2007). It hit on the Martin/St. Lucie county border, five miles from the location where Frances had hit only weeks earlier.

Another caregiver I interviewed said, "We have been lucky since 2005. In 2005, we had Wilma . . . and Katrina crossed the state, but it was only a category 1 when it hit Florida . . . but, they say the oceans are getting warmer and that hurricanes are going to happen more. I don't know. I hope we don't get hit again this year." They didn't. The year 2011 was quiet for Florida. But in 2012, Hurricane Isaac swung close to the Florida coast, causing five tornadoes and loss of power (Berg 2013). There were only five deaths related to Isaac in the United States; however, there were twenty-four directly related deaths in Haiti. Florida was lucky in 2012—but New Jersey and New York were not so fortunate. Later that year, Hurricane Sandy caused $50 billion in damage in the northeastern United States and directly caused 147 deaths across the Atlantic basin (Blake et al. 2013).

The caregiver was correct to be concerned, though. Overwhelming amounts of rigorous, scientific research demonstrate that the carbon concentration of the oceans is increasing, and their temperatures are rising. Warmer oceans mean more frequent and more intense hurricanes with greater storm surge (Trenberth 2007; Wang and Lee 2008; Lin et al. 2012).

THE ELDER HEALTH ECOSYNDEMIC

My own research was on caregiving for someone with Alzheimer's disease during hurricanes in the United States, and most examples given throughout this text are from those who planned for or experienced hurricanes. The lessons illustrated by these examples, however, can be applied to most elders with chronic or temporary illnesses in many countries. Aging populations are growing around the world, though concentrated in developed nations (Cauley 2012). Carbon dioxide emissions do not respect geopolitical boundaries and weather-related disasters are, likewise, not limited to the borders of the United States. What can be different is the cultural framing and how a society chooses to prioritize the underlying, structural issues. In the United States the underlying structural causes create an **ecosyndemic** (which will be discussed in more detail in chapter 2). An ecosyndemic is a complex interaction of health, social conditions, and ecological or ecosocial factors that amplify the negative outcomes of an event (Baer and Singer 2008; Singer 2010). The "eco" in this term refers to the ecosocial. Ecosocial, in turn, is "a configuration of local social environmental conditions (e.g., the social deprivation of living in an impoverished neighborhood) that are the products of class and ethnic inequality" (Singer et al. 2006, 208). Syndemics are the processes of two or more disease pathways that have a synergistic relationship, ultimately amplifying the burden of disease.

The **health conditions** in the ecosyndemic described throughout this book include underlying chronic diseases, disabilities, or general frailty that are correlated with older age. The cultural preference against multigenerational households in the United States is an example of **social conditions** that increase the number of elders with impairments who are living alone or are on low, fixed incomes. The built environment can also amplify the effects; the paucity of public transportation in the United States, for example, can isolate elders or people who cannot drive while also increasing reliance on CO_2-producing motor vehicles. Anthropogenic pollutants are contributing to an increased frequency and severity of extreme weather. Yet there is a powerful minority in society that is funneling economic resources to resist the acceptance of climate science. This resistance to accepting climate change frames the social conditions in which we live. Denying the anthropogenic causes of climate change means that important actors will not act to mitigate the root causes. This aspect is an **ecosocial** factor in this ecosyndemic (e.g., lack of planning for flood surges, intense development in vulnerable coastal areas). Interaction among these three factors—a set of health conditions, a set of social practices and structures of inequality, and a set of environmental changes that reflect human activity—constitute what I call the **Elder Health Ecosyndemic**.

SUMMARY

Chapter 2, "The Elder Health Ecosyndemic," introduces the concept of ecosyndemics, the ecosocial and synergistic interactions of one or more diseases. Ecosyndemics is critical for understanding how, if gone unchecked, global climate change in an aging society can amplify the level of disease and death, especially among the elderly (Gamble et al. 2013; Gamble and Balbus 2016). We are living in a time of climate change, which is exacerbating extreme weather events such as hurricanes and heat waves (chapter 3, "Climate Science and the Ecosocial"). While climatic change has happened in the past, the rapid extremes we are witnessing now are different and, more important, human settlement and subsistence patterns have changed, increasing our vulnerability in several key ways (chapter 4, "Archaeology of Hurricanes"). What complicates things even more is that there are more and more people reaching retirement age, like Betsy and Joe. How we think about older age influences policies and disaster response (chapter 5, "Aging Theory"). It is particularly troubling that vulnerability can be viewed as an acceptable cause of death, an expected loss, rather than an impetus for reducing the vulnerability (Fjord 2010). Older age increases the likelihood of having an age-related disability, which can be exacerbated by a disrupted climate (chapter 6, "Aging, Disability, and Disasters"). How societies choose to respond to such pressures deserves critical examination of ethics because older and disabled populations are implicitly devalued in disaster response (chapter 7, "The Expected Dead: Bioethics, Vulnerability, and Expected Loss"). This is increasingly important as more people are living in hurricane-prone and densely populated areas (chapter 8, "Ecosocial Conditions, Built Environment, and Population Geography"). Long-term care facilities, which many elder populations call home, provide examples of how disaster planning can be done correctly or go horribly wrong (chapter 9, "Social Conditions, Long-Term Care, and Disasters"). Once society accepts that climate change is a legitimate problem that has workable solutions, people can adopt pro-environmental behaviors. With appropriate public health interventions, disaster preparedness in an aging society can be planned for and the risk minimized. It is certainly possible to reduce factors, such as CO_2 production, that exacerbate the rate at which the climate is disrupted. Technology has been developed, urban planning can be adjusted, and consumption patterns altered. However, to do these things takes both an understanding of the underlying problems and the political will to address those problems.

Chapter Two

The Elder Health Ecosyndemic

I never met Lee Marteeny from Everglades City. I read about him in the local newspaper. Lee was seventy-two-years-old when he died after Hurricane Irma hit south Florida. He didn't die in the storm, though. He died days after in Physicians Regional Hospital where he was treated for "respiratory failure and internal bleeding" (Murphy and Cranney 2017, para. 3). Years prior, he had been diagnosed with heart disease and had poor circulation in his legs, which in turn caused sores on his legs (also commonly caused by diabetes). Though they lived in a mobile home in an area predicted to be hit by Hurricane Irma on September 9, 2017, the Marteenys stayed. I don't know why they stayed, but, based my research (including countless interviews, stories, surveys, and personal experience), I can say this: evacuating is expensive, and Everglades City is a lower income fishing community (Murphy and Cranney 2017). Evacuation is also physically taxing, especially for those with mobility limitations. Usually people who do not evacuate for hurricanes are older in age and have successfully survived a hurricane in the past (Eisenman et al. 2007; Christensen, Richey, and Castaneda 2013). Though I did not know Lee or his wife, Lisa, it is possible these factors went through their heads as they weighed the costs and benefits of staying home or evacuating as Hurricane Irma approached.

On Sunday night, Hurricane Irma tore through their community, damaging their trailer, but Lee and Lisa survived. Their trailer was flooded. They lost power and the trailer sustained extensive structural damage, but they remained. The Monday after the hurricane hit, the temperature reached 92°F but felt hotter because the air was humid (*New York Times* 2017). Though the floors, walls, and bedding were damp, the Marteenys slept in the trailer because there was no "shelter or temporary housing in town" (Murphy and Cranney 2017). Even if hotel rooms had been available, they might not have been able to afford to rent one.

For five days, they tried to clean and sleep in their home. By Thursday, the sores on Lee's legs began to turn black after wading through the flood waters, indicating an infection (Murphy and Cranney 2017). On Friday, he was in so much pain they called an ambulance to transport him to the hospital. That night, he was in respiratory distress. By Saturday, he was dead.

Lee's death is likely the result of a complex interaction of physical, social, economic, and environmental factors that made him more vulnerable to certain diseases. Many diseases associated with older age, such as congestive heart failure, have a synergistic relationship with other diseases, like diabetes. The effect of one disease can amplify the effects of another, creating what Merrill Singer has called "a perfect epidemiological storm" of vulnerability (Singer 2008). The vulnerability to age-related diseases is amplified by being of a lower socioeconomic status, which can limit access to healthier foods and safe housing and potentially access to preventative medical care.

The resources in the community in which Lee lived were limited. The lack of resources may have also limited options when faced with an intense risk, such as Hurricane Irma. They could have gone to a shelter, but there are barriers, real and imagined, to access to them. For example, it is unclear from the newspaper articles if the Marteenys had a car.

Age, heat, underlying chronic illnesses, poor housing conditions, amplified by the disaster, all contributed to Lee's ultimate death. As the climate grows more disrupted, critical events that amplify risk of death and injury are likely to increase. As a warming climate decreases air quality, the conditions of age-related illnesses and disability are simultaneously made worse. As climate change fuels stronger storms, people with these illnesses and disabilities will have a more difficult time preparing, responding, and recovering. As Maureen Coyle explains:

> An elderly person may, but need not be, extremely vulnerable: An individual who is elderly and lives with others in a safe, clean, climate-controlled space with a dependable food supply is a lot less vulnerable than the older individual who is economically insecure, who is ill, cognitively impaired, who lives in isolation and is very vulnerable indeed to the impacts of climate change. (2015, 80)

SYNDEMICS

Some diseases or "co-infections" can hasten the spread and progression of or exacerbate the level of disability of another disease. Tuberculosis and HIV are examples of diseases that have this kind of synergistic relationship (Singer et al. 2006; Singer and Clair 2003). These diseases tend to have a bidirectional relationship (the damage they cause is enhanced by the presence of the other disease). Another example of this kind of potentially lethal synergy is the relationship that can develop between influenza viruses (or "the flu") and pneumococcus bacteria (which are the cause of pneumonia) (Singer 2009). The frail elderly are especially susceptible to such upper respiratory interaction co-infections (Fulop et al. 2010).

Medical anthropologist Merrill Singer explains that the biomechanisms driving this synergy are as follows: (1) the influenza virus can damage or weaken the lungs, and it can lower the body's ability to mobilize its immune system, which can (2) allow for the pneumococcus to invade the body (Singer 2013, 99). This synergistic relationship results in "excess mortality from secondary bacterial pneumonia during influenza epidemics" (Singer 2013, 99). In other words, these two diseases "work together" to become more lethal than they would be alone. The effects of their interaction are not just additive, they are multiplicative.

Syndemics is a term related to the **synergy** between two diseases, but syndemics also involves a layer of social interaction; syndemics describes how human biology and social status (often, as noted below, mediated by the environment) can influence the progression of a disease (by bringing diseases into interaction). Social conditions, like poverty, are linked with malnutrition, stress, trauma, and toxic exposure, which can weaken the body's immune system and make it more vulnerable to infectious diseases (Baer and Singer 2008; Singer 2009). As a biosocial theoretical model, syndemics critically examines how poverty and social relationships generally (or lack thereof) can hasten the progression of a disease, and, as well, can lead to the clustering of diseases that then are afforded the opportunity to adversely interact.

Unequal social relations (variously expressed as impoverishment, stigmatization, structural violence, discrimination, and marginalization) result in exposure to adverse living and working conditions in subordinate populations, which, in turn, promote the clustering of both infectious and noninfectious diseases and both organic and behavioral disorders, while weakening the body's capacity for responding to disease challenges (Singer 2013). The number and nature of an interaction and the social conditions that promote them significantly shape the burden of syndemic disease in a population.

Environmental factors can also amplify underlying social conditions, which can expose economically disadvantaged individuals to a greater duration and number of hazards. For example, respiratory-related syndemics (like the flu and pneumonia) can be greatly exacerbated by changes in the environment resulting from poor air quality (Singer 2013). Respiratory health-related disease interactions can be immediate (triggering asthma attacks) or delayed (causing damage to the lungs over time). This has led researchers to carefully consider syndemics within the context of climate change. Baer and Singer called this an **ecosyndemic**, which considers how global warming can magnify or speed up a syndemic (Baer and Singer 2008, 2014; Singer 2010, 2013).

ECOSYNDEMICS

The concept of ecosyndemics is helpful for understanding how, if gone unchecked, global climate change in an aging society can amplify the level of disease and death we are likely to see, especially among the elderly. It adds yet another layer to the synergistic manifestation of disease and illness. In addition to factors such as poverty, ecosyndemics also draws attention to how changing environmental factors resulting from a warmer climate can exacerbate health problems (Baer and Singer 2008).

Keeping with the example of influenza viruses and pneumococcus bacteria, the symptoms of this syndemic disease (primarily affecting the lungs) can be made worse by man-made toxins in the environment. Not everyone has the same exposure to these pollutants: individuals who work outdoors, such as landscapers or street vendors, tend to have higher exposures and also tend to come from lower socioeconomic backgrounds (Singer 2013). Unchecked pollution in Shanghai, China, for example, has led to unprecedented levels of respiratory illnesses, especially among those who are economically disadvantaged (Singer 2013).

SYNDEMICS: THE DUNMORES AND THE MARTEENYS

As in Betsy and Joe Dunmore's example from chapter 1, the greater number of older individuals living in coastal areas can make them especially vulnerable to an increase in the number and intensity of hurricanes. Joe had an illness that might have impaired his ability to recognize his need for fluids in the extreme heat after a hurricane. It was Betsy, his wife and caregiver, who assisted him with his hydration and kept him safe. After the cascading events of multiple hurricanes, and consequent physical strain, Betsy's health was also compromised (though not fatally), as exemplified by her high blood pressure. Betsy and Joe's social and financial standing helped them to weather the storm and the associated challenges of the hurricanes. Individuals of lower economic status might be less able to handle the blows of multiple hurricanes. Thus, Betsy and Joe had means of transportation to evacuate the area and funds to pay for a hotel, which was not the case for many older black residents affected by Hurricane Katrina in New Orleans. They also demonstrate a very different social situation than the Marteenys, who indicated that they could not afford a $900 annual insurance policy on the mobile home. Mobile homes remain one of the most vulnerable structures in the face of hurricanes (Kusenbach and Taylor 2012).

ECOSYNDEMICS: CLIMATE CHANGE AND TURMOIL

According to NASA, the (2008) definition of global warming is "the increase in Earth's average surface temperature due to rising levels of greenhouse gases" (Conway 2008). NOAA describes "climate change" as the best term to describe the alterations to Earth's climate because, in addition to rising temperatures, there are changes in precipitation patterns and sea levels (Mauritsen and Pincus 2017; Elert and Lemonick 2012). Other terms, such as "global weirdness," have been presented as a more accessible and accurate term, drawing attention to the unexpected, more extreme outcomes of a warming climate (Elert and Lemonick 2012). The concept of "climate turmoil" is presented by Baer and Singer, who argue that climate change is not the best term to describe the alterations, some of which, like ocean rise or vector-borne disease spread, are not measures of the climate changing but are consequences of such change: "hence, to capture all the complexities and their profound effects, we use the term 'climate turmoil' to describe the diverse impacts of climate change" (2014).

This terminology captures the result of a warming climate: the turmoil experienced by humans responding to impacts. Singer summarizes that "global warming is driving increases in frequency of intense storms, the length of droughts, the gravity of heat waves, the severity of flooding, the toll of forest fires, the water level of the oceans, the melting of the ice caps, the production of allergens and the graphical range of climate-sensitive vectors of infectious disease" and, I add, is increasing the stress placed on older bodies (2009, 190). The development of age-related impairments can make it more difficult to respond to intense storms, floods, wildfires, or other disasters. Increased allergens, including those produced from the smoke of wildfires, are more difficult for people with upper-respiratory illnesses or cardiopulmonary disease (COPD) to tolerate (Allen 2015; Gamble et al. 2013).

Understanding the ecosynemics around age and climage change means understanding how climate change is constructed in the public sphere. Climate change is a politically charged subject, but there is scientific consensus that (1) CO_2 levels are increasing in the atmosphere and in the oceans (Mauritsen and Pincus 2017; Elert and Lemonick 2012); (2) CO_2 levels are increasing because of human causes, including an increase in the burning of fossil fuels over the last 150 years (Knowlton et al. 2011; Solomon et al. 2007); (3) as a result of climate change, we can expect to see disruption of familiar climate patterns and we will endure stronger enviornmental hazards (Trenberth 2007, 2012; Wright, Knutson, and Smith 2015; Baptiste 2017; Emanuel 2005); and (4) oceans are warming, which drives an increase in the number and intensity of hurricanes ("Global Warming and Hurricanes" 2017).

In spite of scientific concensus, there is vast popular confusion surrounding the ideas of global warming and climate change (Clynes 2012; Oreskes and Conway 2010b; Hulac 2016). Denial rhetoric is important because it is often brought into climate change debates and is sometimes used to intentionally obfuscate the issues (which will be discussed further in chapter 6). There is very little evidence to suggest that global warming is not caused by human actions. Of all the research on climate, only 3 percent of published papers cast doubt on whether the changes are anthropogenic in nature (Benestad et al. 2016). Those papers were enough to create an illusion of vast controversy within the science community (when in fact there really wasn't one). In 2017, the research casting doubt on the anthropogenic causes of climate change was reviewed again, highlighting flaws in research design and analysis (Foley 2017).

Multiple public health concerns are associated with a warming climate: increasing extreme storm severity, spread of vector- and water-borne infectious diseases, frequency of mold-caused disease, frequency of allergies, and heat-related health effects (Shultz, Russell, and Espinel 2005). The upsurge in ecosyndemics suggests a need for planned public health interventions.

Higher CO_2 concentrations in the atmosphere means that the oceans heat faster and retain heat longer. The warmer the ocean temperatures, the more likely tropical cyclones will form (Emanuel 2005, 2012; Knutson et al. 2010, 2015). The expected increased number of hurricanes triggered by global warming is likely to affect people who are older or come from lower socioeconomic backgrounds disproportionately (Lupton 1993, 425). For example, even though people over the age of sixty-five made up less than 12 percent of the pre-Katrina New Orleans population, they accounted for 64 percent of all storm-related deaths. According to Brunkard and colleagues, "Older black people in Orleans Parish, particularly men, were disproportionately represented [in the death records] relative to their underlying population distribution" (Brunkard, Namulanda, and Ratard 2008, 7). This pattern continued with Hurricane Sandy. In total, there were 117 deaths as a result of Hurricane Sandy; the average age of those who died was sixty ("Deaths Associated with Hurricane Sandy" 2013). Older individuals are more likely to have underlying chronic diseases, which can be triggered or exacerbated during weather extremes and related power outages. Older individuals who come from minority populations and have lower income are even more at risk. I argue that the intersection of (1) climate-driven hurricane severity and (2) increasing incidence of entwined age-related diseases operate as an ecosyndemic that is likely to become even more deadly as the climate becomes more tumultuous.

PUBLIC HEALTH AND RISK

Risk determinations are based on mathematical possibilities and social interest: "In dealing with civilization's risks, the sciences have always abandoned their foundation of experimental logic and made a polygamous marriage with business, politics, and ethics" (Beck 1986, 29). Risk, in its most common usage, is a measure of danger. Deborah Lupton, an anthropologist and public health professional, notes that, in its original usage, "'Risk' is neutral, referring to probability, or the mathematical likelihood of an event occurring" (1993). The risk of an event occurring could therefore be related to either a positive or negative outcome, as in "the risk of winning the lottery" (Lupton 1999, 81). In public health, "risk" is used as a synonym for "danger."

Public health campaigns are an attempt to help people assess and reduce risks to their health. There are many complex reasons why people are not very good at assessing risks, especially when it comes to weather-related events like hurricanes:

1. People may lack information about risk or how to prepare (access).
2. They may not understand the information or how to use it (comprehension).
3. They may not have the means to properly prepare (socioeconomic factors).
4. They may not trust the people or entities that are providing them information about risk (risk perception). (Sorensen and Sorensen 2007)

Two theorists, Ulrich Beck and Anthony Giddens, have argued that the modern era has changed how citizens view, understand, and respond to risk. While Beck argues that there has been an actual increase in hazards, such as more diseases, higher chance of biological warfare or other deadly weapons, and more environmental events, with modernity, Giddens counters that it only appears this way because risk is more visible (1990). (A hazard is an exposure to something that has the potential to harm. A hurricane is, technically, a hazard. It only becomes a disaster if it has a deleterious impact on some populations. A hazard carries risk for those exposed to it.) What is important, however, is that both theorists agree that individuals in the modern era tend to be hyperaware of the risks they face, due in part to public health campaigns and the media. This state of hyperawareness of risk is referred to as a "risk society."

Although people may be hyperaware of risks, they might not act to reduce all risks. Indeed, the sheer number of risks that a single person faces daily can be overwhelming: too much sun can cause skin cancer, the air one breathes might be polluted and cause illness, packaged foods might contain dyes and genetically modified organisms (GMOs). To a large extent, people rely on governmental regulations to help them vet risks. For example, people may trust that the Food and Drug Administration (FDA) has scrutinized the food they eat.

Giddens and Beck, however, point to an increased distrust in government officials, scientists, and public health officials who, at times, provide conflicting or inaccurate information. Prior to Hurricane Katrina, for example, many residents of Louisiana and Mississippi had either survived previous hurricanes despite government-issued hurricane warnings or had evacuated for a hurricane that, in hindsight, they did not feel posed a threat. These experiences influenced how they responded to warnings and evacuation orders when Hurricane Katrina approached. Ultimately, it can be difficult for individuals to determine when they are at risk enough to require action when threatened with a natural disaster, such as a hurricane. Indeed, research has shown that older people are less likely to evacuate when a hurricane threatens their area than younger people (Eisenman et al. 2007, 2009; Dash and Gladwin 2007; Christensen, Richey, and Castaneda 2013).

Public health campaigns are conducted to warn the public about risks to their health. If armed with this knowledge, people will avoid these risks. Lupton distinguishes between two kinds of risks: (1) environmental (such as toxic waste, radiation, genetic predisposition, or a hurricane), over which the individual has little control; and (2) risk behaviors, resulting from lifestyle choices, such as smoking or choosing to evacuate for a hurricane (Nichter 2003). The second category assumes that the risk is something over which the individual has control, while the former does not. For instance, during Hurricane Katrina, people were frequently blamed for not evacuating in spite of warnings. Though they did not have control over the hurricane, it was assumed that people had control over their location during the hurricane. This is much like when an individual who eats a high-fat diet is blamed for having a heart attack, even if access to healthier foods is limited by geography and income.

Public health professionals and anthropologists (such as Lupton and Nichter) argue that individuals must believe that a threat actually exists (risk identification) and believe that protection is needed (risk assessment) before they are willing to engage in risk-reducing behaviors, such as making a disaster plan (Guion, Scammon, and Borders 2007). For individuals to work through these steps, they must believe that the information provided by the government and experts is valid and that the safeguards they depend upon will be in place. For example, citizens must believe that a hurricane warning is valid and poses a true risk to their well-being to heed such a warning. Those who decide to evacuate to shelters must first believe that the government will adequately provide a safe and reliable sanctuary. According to Giddens, this trust may not exist, and when individuals are skeptical of the so-called experts, they may choose to ignore the risk entirely (Giddens 1990). If citizens do not trust the experts who assess the direction of a hurricane and its likely severity, they may not identify it as a risk. Beck likewise contends that a condition of modernity is that science no longer has "a monopoly on rationality," and, as a consequence, "there is no [universally accepted] expert on risk" (1986, 29).

Anthropologist Mark Nichter found that many individuals do not perceive themselves at risk, even if statistics indicate that they are at risk (2003). A major role of public health professionals (including emergency managers) is to inform the public of their level of risk and convince them to adopt risk-reducing strategies, such as compiling a disaster kit (Guion, Scammon, and Borders 2007). If public health officials cannot convince the population that hurricane preparedness is important, then it is unlikely that citizens will comply with efforts or pressure from elected officials to legislate additional mitigation measures. From a public health perspective, an important challenge is to convince the public that disaster preparedness is a priority among all other risks of daily life, especially outside hurricane season. They might also make other choices that would reduce their risk of being affected by a chronic illness.

In the following section, theories are presented on why people might not respond to emergencies in the way public health professionals (or the popular media) would like.

DISASTERS AND VULNERABILITY

According to Beck, "Poverty attracts an unfortunate abundance of risks. By contrast, the wealthy (in income, power or education) can purchase safety and freedom from risk" (1986, 35).

Disasters do not have the same impact on everyone in society; there are disproportionate impacts on people with lower socioeconomic standing. This is a function of social, political, and economic status (which is why critical medical anthropology is a valuable framework).

The concept of "vulnerability" is central to the understanding of disproportionate disaster impacts. Populations such as those with lower socioeconomic status, marginalized minority groups, those with preexisting health conditions, and the elderly tend to be more vulnerable to the deleterious effects of disasters (Cutter 2003; Phifer, Kaniasty, and Norris 1988; Phifer 1990; Morrow 1999; Hutton 2008). Most of the casualties of Hurricane Katrina in 2005 fit into one or all of these categories (Jenkins, Laska, and Williamson 2007; Rothman and Brown 2006). The concept of vulnerability in disaster research refers to certain subsets of the population that bear an undue burden of the impact due to their lower socioeconomic status, age, or preexisting health conditions. Vulnerability is defined by Wisner et al. as

> The characteristics of a person or group and their situation that influence their capacity to anticipate, cope with, resist and recover from the impact of a natural hazard (an extreme natural event or process). It involves a combination of factors that determine the degree to which someone's life, livelihood, property and other assets are put at risk by a discrete and identifiable event (or series or "cascade" of such events) in nature and in society. (2004, 11)

The elderly experience disproportionately high levels of poverty in many countries around the world, which in turn makes it difficult for them to respond in the face of disaster hazards (Fernandez et al. 2002; Hutton 2008; Carnes, Staats, and Willcox 2014). Furthermore, as elderly populations have a higher incidence of debilitation and disability than younger populations, they may have more physical barriers to appropriate preparations and response to a threat of a hurricane. As Wisner et al. elaborate, "Debilitation and disability mean that people have less time to invest in protecting themselves from other hazards" (2004, 29).

The ways in which a hazard impacts a population are determined by several structural factors, including socioeconomic status, minority group membership, and age (Singer 2009, 190). The existence of preparations and plans for mitigation can also impact the outcomes of a hazard event and ultimately determine whether it will be labeled a "disaster" or simply bad weather. The public health impacts of hurricanes are outlined by Shultz, Russell, and Espinel as the following: storm-related mortality, injury, infectious disease, psychosocial effects, displacement and homelessness, damage to the health care infrastructure, disruption of public health services, transformation of critical ecosystems, social dislocation, loss of jobs and livelihood, and economic crisis (2005, 21). An increase in communicable diseases after hurricanes is important to note, especially regarding vulnerable populations (such as the poor and the elderly).

They also explain that a person (or group's) resilience, sometimes defined as the capacity to recover one's livelihood, is considered an integral part of the concept of vulnerability. Perhaps a better definition of resilience is the one presented by the Intergovernmental Panel on Climate Change (IPCC): "the ability of a system and its component parts to anticipate, absorb, accommodate, or recover from the effects of a hazardous event in a timely and efficient manner, including through ensuring the preservation, restoration, or improvement of its essential basic structures and functions" (Barros et al. 2014, 5). For elders, preparing for, responding to, and recovering from a disaster can be much more difficult than for younger people (Hutton 2008).

SUMMARY

Disease and illness operates within social and ecological environments. The concept of syndemics comes from critical medical anthropology to explain the synergistic nature of some diseases, which are then amplified by social structures. An ecosyndemic considers the syndemic within its environment. The building blocks of an ecosyndemic are the health, social, and environmental conditions. Climate change and pollution are an underlying factor in many syndemics and remain a factor in the Elder Health Syndemic. The latter part of the life span correlates with the body being less resilient to temperature extremes. As climate change is making temperatures more volatile, morbidity and mortality are likely to increase in a synergistic manner.

Chapter Three

Climate Science and the Ecosocial

"I have a bad feeling about this year. . . . It has been so hot this winter. Very hot. Where I come from [Puerto Rico] we worry when it is a hot winter like this" (professional caregiver, Palm Beach County, 2011, as cited in Christensen 2012). While working with caregivers in West Palm Beach, Florida, in 2010–2011, only two of the thirty people I formally interviewed brought up the temperature of the oceans or the concept of climate change as we discussed hurricane risk and preparedness. Climate change was not a point of discussion during the nine months of participant observation, working with formal caregivers in adult day care centers and with informal, family caregivers. It was not a targeted part of my research either; however, in qualitative research, the topics that remain unaddressed can be as interesting as those that are explicitly discussed. Why didn't more participants make the connection between hurricanes and a disrupted climate? Though I did not ask about climate change, it is noteworthy that so few people intuitively connected the links between hurricane damages and a disrupted climate. Scientific studies support the fact that a warmer winter can mean that the oceans heat up earlier in the season, and warmer oceans are more likely to cause hurricanes, as the nurse quoted above suggested (Trenberth 2007; Knutson et al. 2010).

We were lucky in 2011, as a hurricane did not hit Florida. The following year, Hurricane Sandy breezed by the state of Florida and inundated the coast of the northeastern United States, including in New Jersey and New York. There were some connections to sea level rise in the media discussions of the damage caused by Hurricane Sandy (Gibbs and Holloway 2013; Subaiya et al. 2014).

It is perhaps unsurprising that the people with whom I worked were not eager to connect hurricanes to climate change because there have been targeted misinformation campaigns to sow confusion about the topic (Milman 2017; Hansen et al. 2015). Embracing or rejecting the science behind climate change has become almost tribal in the United States, falling along party lines (Dressler and Parson 2010; Jylhä et al. 2016). Internationally, rejecting climate change is highly correlated with evangelical Christian religious affiliation (Greeley 1993; Schultz, Zelezny, and Dalrymple 2000; Smith and Leiserowitz 2013; Morrison, Duncan, and Parton 2015). Another study found that conservative white males tend to deny the anthropogenic effects of climate change (McCright and Dunlap 2011).

The rapidly changing climate and the related disruption of weather patterns are the ecological foundation in the **Elder Health Ecosyndemic**. What follows is an abbreviated summary of the scientific consensus on changing climate across the globe, which ultimately affects all living things.

CRITICAL MEDICAL ANTHROPOLOGY AND CLIMATE SCIENCE

Critical medical anthropology is concerned with connecting macro-level political economics with cultural influences on health. From an anthropological standpoint, the controversy surrounding climate change is of interest because it has caused confusion among lay populations, which stalls needed mitigation on a political level. There are many political-economic reasons for denying climate change, including the potential regulation of polluting organizations (Elsasser and Dunlap 2012; Hulm 2009). Even if climate change were to be widely accepted as an urgent issue, it is unlikely that the companies that profit from the extraction and/or burning of fossil fuels would swiftly volunteer to reduce their pollutants or advocate for a reduced dependence (at least not without a decrease in demand). Instead, the government would have to step in and regulate these businesses, likely by imposing financial sanctions on polluters (Bartlett, Naranjo, and Plugis 2017; Singer and Baer 2009). The increased cost would decrease the large profits currently enjoyed by their shareholders.

The increased cost of fossil fuel dependence is passed on to the consumer, those of us who are dependent on the automobile for transportation in the suburbs, for example. Even food would become more expensive, as transportation of produce is largely done via diesel-fueled trucks on the highway. Americans would have to reprioritize their consumption patterns, which would be a painful process, especially for those with lower incomes. Indeed, when gas prices rise, there is often a highly publicized outcry (Blustein and Timberg 2005).

This would not be all bad, however. It is possible that increased gas prices would spur a demand for cleaner technology and efficient public transportation options. Even car manufacturers, such as former General Motors CEO Dan Akerson, called for a tax on gasoline that would increase demand for smaller, more efficient cars (which they are mandated to provide, even if they are not in high demand when gas prices are lower) (Busse, Knittel, and Zettelmeyer 2012). Alan Mulally, the former CEO of Ford, has also supported a gasoline tax (*Wall Street Journal* 2009).

While some corporate owners support further regulation, others find government intervention to be unnecessary at best, tyrannical and oppressive at worst. Some view government regulation as a personal assault on their ability to extract the most potential from their financial endeavors. When a person's portfolio shows fewer returns due to regulations, he or she might feel that their well-being is threatened. Certainly, it is easier to value immediate gratification over potential environmental degradation, although the longer-term consequences for the inhabitants of the planet could be disastrous.

When President George W. Bush first took office in 2001, he openly acknowledged that he withdrew the United States from the Kyoto Protocol on limiting CO_2 emissions because it would have placed regulations on businesses and had a negative impact on the economy (Hulm 2009; Oreskes and Conway 2010a). Later in his administration's tenure, there was outright questioning and suppression of science. There was a deliberate misinformation campaign about climate change (Donaghy et al. 2007; "Agencies Control Scientists' Contacts with the Media" 2004). These strategies continue in some individual states, such as Florida under the leadership of Governor Rick Scott (Korten 2015).

As happened with the (so-called) debate surrounding the impact of secondhand cigarette smoke, powerful companies have worked to obscure scientific facts to maintain their profits (Singer and Baer 2009). The connection between cigarette smoke and the climate change debates is stronger than one might realize: it was the same physicists (Fred Seitz and Fred Singer) who spearheaded the attack on the connection between secondhand cigarette smoke and cancer in the late 1970s and 1980s and who also engineered the attack on global warming scientists in the late 1990s (Oreskes and Conway 2010a).

In the early 2000s, the Bush administration embraced the aura of doubt created by Seitz and Singer, even though these two men were World War II physicists who had not themselves done original work on tobacco smoke or climate science; they had helped engineer the atomic bomb, and as a result were politically well connected and later helped to administer funding from cigarette companies and conservative think tanks to researchers who could potentially (but failed to) disprove the link between cancer and cigarette smoke (Oreskes and Conway 2010a).

The Bush administration instituted a policy that forbade scientists working at NASA or NOAA from speaking to the media about climate change. Chris Mooney, a science writer, followed several high-profile weather scientists at international conferences in 2005 and 2006 (2007). He specifically focused on the relationship between a warmer climate and the increasing severity of cyclonic storms such as hurricanes. It was during these years that the Bush administration began to limit press access to the climate scientists working for the federal government (in the National Oceanic and Atmospheric Administration). Mooney also notes that there was a "historically rooted and methodologically grounded rivalry between two groups of scientists studying the same meteorological phenomenon from very different vantage points" (2007, 12). These methodological differences were spun and exploited by the Bush administration to create further doubt. They created an effective campaign against the climate change concept.

After the Bush administration, there were eight years of the Obama administration, which prioritized climate change and adopted science-based policies. Following this, the Trump administration has returned to the stance of denial set by the Bush/Cheney administration. If climate change is denied as a true problem, then attention and resources will not be allocated to address it. It allows for the status quo to continue: dependency on fossil fuels, their extraction, and development without attention to public transportation—thus forcing a continued reliance on motor vehicles. The primary sources of CO_2 will continue to be pumped into the atmosphere, degrading environmental conditions and making humans, especially the elderly, sicker.

FACTORS, CAUSES, INFLUENCES ON CLIMATE DISRUPTION AND TURMOIL

Climate change does not mean that every year will be hotter than the last, nor will the whole earth warm at the same rate. The Arctic and Antarctic poles, for example, are warming faster than other places on Earth. The poles, with their ice caps, usually act as a giant mirror, reflecting the sun's heat back into the atmosphere (Wadhams 2013; Brumfield and Todd 2014; Kim et al. 2014; Petoukhov and Semenov 2010). As the ice caps melt, the mirror becomes smaller. The heat no longer reflected away from Earth is now absorbed. More heat makes the ice caps melt even faster. The is called a positive (warming) feedback loop, because the heat causes the ice caps to melt, which means there is less ice to reflect away heat, and in turn, melts them even faster. Scientists are observing this phenomenon in action: though the glaciers and ice caps have been shrinking since about 1850, the rate of loss in Greenland is rapidly increasing (Corell 2008; Wadhams 2013). Decreases in sea ice (due to warmer climates) can bring about colder winters in northern continents, due to a weakened polar vortex (Kim et al. 2014). The winter of 2014 in the US Midwest is an example of this phenomenon.

Melting ice also causes sea levels to rise, which threatens coastal cities, especially during hurricane-caused storm surges (Corell 2008; Lin et al. 2012; Woodruff, Irish, and Camargo 2013). Sea levels are, indeed, rising. In 2012, the sea levels were eight inches higher than they were in 1900 (Berkman and Vylegzhanin 2013). It is perhaps counterintuitive, but the sea does not rise the same amount everywhere; currents can cause the sea level to rise faster in some places than in other places, such as in Miami, Florida (Wdowinski et al. 2016; Valle-Levinson, Dutton, and Martin 2017).

Another source of warming feedback is CO_2. When the temperature is warmer, the oceans absorb less CO_2 than they do when it is colder (Lackner et al. 2012). This means that more CO_2 is trapped in the atmosphere instead. More CO_2 in the atmosphere traps more heat, causing the oceans to become even warmer. In addition, warmer temperatures cause more evaporation from the oceans and other bodies of water. Water vapor in the atmosphere also traps heat and is far more abundant than CO_2 (Held and Soden 2000).

There are multiple complex players that influence the climate, but CO_2 is the most problematic because it stays in the atmosphere for a prolonged period and it also accumulates in the oceans (Lackner et al. 2012; Fearnside 2012). Carbon dioxide is only part of the problem that contributes to global climate change. Nitrogen and oxygen are the two most abundant gases in the atmosphere. Water vapor is the third most abundant. Carbon dioxide is a problem because humans are adding it to the atmosphere, causing oceans to warm, adding water vapor to the atmosphere, and trapping even more heat (Miller et al. 2011). This cycle, or feedback loop, continues. As CO_2 increases and the climate gets warmer, more water will evaporate and trap more heat, causing the warming feedback described above. Water vapor amplifies the warming from CO_2 emissions (Held and Soden 2000). If we can control CO_2 in the atmosphere, we might be able to control the amount of water vapor in the atmosphere and slow the rate of ice cap melt. Global leaders have not yet succeeded in doing this.

Methane is also a common greenhouse gas, but it breaks down quicker in the atmosphere than CO_2. Unlike methane, CO_2 can stay in the atmosphere for thousands of years and continue to trap heat ("WMO Provisional Statement" 2017). This means that, even if we were to immediately stop all fossil fuel emissions, the planet would continue to warm for many years to come. A quarter of the CO_2 in the atmosphere comes from fossil fuels and it is increasing. More feedback is created as humans cut down the rain forests; the destruction of rain forests means that the natural cycle of CO_2 removal is disrupted.

OCEANS AND CLIMATE: PACIFIC DECADAL OSCILLATION, EL NIÑO / LA NIÑA (ENSO)

The oceans have an ongoing effect on weather patterns. A Reuters headline in January 2018 read: "Earth Sweltered Again in 2017: Hottest Year without an El Nino" (Doyle). The article explained that though 2017 was only the third hottest year on record, it was the warmest on record without the added heat caused by the weather pattern called El Niño. The El Niño event occurs every few years, though it is irregular, defying a pattern. When it occurs, it "releases heat from the tropical Pacific Ocean into the atmosphere" creating wetter, hotter conditions (Doyle 2018, paragraph 5).

The World Meteorological Organization (WMO) explained that El Niño events tend to raise global temperatures above the average of the drier, cooler La Niña years ("WMO Provisional Statement" 2017). These events tend to cause flooding in the state of California and in Peru, while droughts ravaged the Papua New Guinea highlands (Jacka 2009). During La Niña, droughts are common in California and Peru (Fagan 2004). With the addition of greenhouse gases, models suggest that the extremes will become even greater (Cai et al. 2015).

This means that the pendulum that naturally swings from wet and warm to dry and cold is likely to swing further out to the extremes.

DISASTERS RELATED TO CLIMATE CHANGE:
LOADING THE DICE

In the winter of 2014, snowstorms blanketed both New England and the southeast as far south as Florida (Brumfield and Todd 2014). Japan was hit with extremely cold weather ("Deadly Winter Weather Paralyzes Japan" 2014). During this same winter, however, California experienced a drought and Vancouver, Canada, was unseasonably warm (Brumfield and Todd 2014). The UK experienced heavy rain that caused flooding of the Thames. Meanwhile, in Sochi, Russia, where the 2014 winter Olympics were held, snow machines were used to adequately cover the slopes for skiing (Brumfield and Todd 2014).

Climate disruption means that areas used by humans at one point in time might no longer be suitable if the climate shifts. Some areas are likely to experience conditions such as floods, droughts, heat waves, cold snaps (blizzards), and increased number and intensity of hurricanes. While it is difficult to attribute a single disaster event to a changing climate, scientists can "calculate whether climate change has tipped the odds in favor of such events happening—whether the coin you're flipping has become slightly loaded in favor of tails, for example" (Elert and Lemonick. 2012, 117). The influences of climate change made the 2003 European heat wave at least twice as likely to occur as it would otherwise have been without a warmer planet (Beniston and Diaz 2004; Della-Marta et al. 2007; Huber and Gulledge 2011). Scientists have also been able to calculate the increased probability of stronger cyclonic storms (i.e., hurricanes, tropical cyclones, typhoons) (Trenberth 2007, 2012; Knutson et al. 2010; Reed et al. 2015).

Heat Waves

Heat waves are defined as an extended number of days and nights where the temperature is above average. It is easy to understand how a warming world can increase the frequency of heat waves. Global temperature averages have risen 2.4°F (1.3°C) from 1880 to 2016 (Stott, Stone, and Allen 2004). According to Gamble, the predicted increase in heat waves will have dire effects on older populations (Gamble et al. 2013; Gamble and Balbus 2016). Areas most vulnerable to heat waves are in higher latitudes, where people and the built environment are less adapted to prolonged heat, especially in large metropolitan areas (Luber and McGeehin 2008; Mann et al. 2017).

Droughts: Water Access and Food Production

The IPCC carefully states that "globally, the area affected by drought has likely increased since the 1970's" (Sauerborn and Ebi 2012). They are cautious in their statement because it is difficult to collectively measure global rainfall and drought indicators. Drought can cause localized food scarcity, especially in areas where people depend on subsistence farming. Even in industrialized areas, such as California, drought can have detrimental effects on food production. Even in a warming climate, drought is not expected to be worldwide; in fact, as droughts prevail in some areas, heavy precipitation will dominate in others. According to Huber and Gulledge, "Observed trends in heat, heavy precipitation, and drought in different places are consistent with global warming" (2011). When human population density was lower, and populations were less tied to agriculture, movement from one place to a more hospitable climate was more likely (Fagan 2004, 2008). Boundaries and terms like "illegal aliens" did not prevent access to other land, climate, or resources.

Wildfires

Drought can also lead to an increase in wildfires, as they dry vegetation (Abatzoglou and Williams 2016). As heat dries out wood, it becomes easy tinder if lightning strikes in the area. The most common type of fire is a "surface fire," which "burns along the floor of a forest, moving slowly and killing or damaging trees" (Landesman 2005, 23). This means that, like a hurricane, there is often some warning, allowing for populations to evacuate. When wood burns, it also releases large amounts of CO_2 into the atmosphere and degrades air quality, which can exacerbate health conditions for some populations (Schneider et al. 2011). Areas damaged by wildfire can lead to erosion of the soil. Without the roots of living vegetation in place on mountain sides, lower-lying areas are at risk of mudslides (Noji 2005).

Floods

It may seem counterintuitive, but droughts are linked with more frequent flooding. When the ground is drier, it may not absorb the water as quickly, causing flash floods (Huber and Gulledge 2011). In a warming climate, water evaporates from the oceans and is also pulled from the soil. As a result, land will tend to be drier, but when the rain or snow does come, there is more water vapor stored up in the atmosphere, so precipitation should become heavier (Kundzewicz et al. 2014).

Blizzards

The polar vortex is impacted by warming poles, which causes changes in high and low pressure systems. During colder times, the cold air that circulates in the poles remains tightly coiled. As it warms, the circulation unravels and cold air from the poles drops farther south (Francis and Vavrus 2012). In addition, as overall warmer temperatures tend to evaporate more water from the Gulf of Mexico and Atlantic Ocean, the amount of atmospheric moisture available to fuel winter storms, such as nor'easters, has been increasing (Huber and Gulledge 2011).

Air Quality

Burning fossil fuels not only has an abstract impact on the atmosphere, it can have a localized impact on air quality, which in turn can be detrimental to human health (Singer 2013; Baer 2016; Gamble et al. 2013). Exposure to poor air quality is a problem in both developing and industrialized nations. In the former, wood burning in poorly ventilated areas can cause exposure. In the latter, dependence on motor vehicles and factory production can cause elevated levels of pollution (Schneider et al. 2011). In either case, the impact on human health can be detrimental, especially among individuals with cardiovascular disease (Pillemer et al. 2011) . Air quality is further degraded by drought-related wildfires, which can produce smoke that irritates the lungs.

Increased Intensity of Hurricanes

Warmer oceans are caused by higher CO_2 concentrations in the atmosphere (Trenberth 2007; Emanuel 2005, 2007). This in turn fuels stronger hurricanes (Knutson et al. 2010; Kossin, Olander, and Knapp 2013). The Power Dissipation Index (PDI) "is an aggregate measure of Atlantic Hurricane activity, combining frequency, intensity, and duration of hurricanes in a single index" ("Global Warming and Hurricanes" 2013, part 2, para. 1). As such, the PDI captures more information about storms over time than the Saffir-Simpson wind scale (which indicates the destructive potential of a cyclonic storm, primarily based on wind strength). Emanuel has documented strong correlations between PDI over time and increasing tropical Atlantic sea-surface temperatures (SST); both the temperature of the ocean (SST) and the destructiveness of storms over time have increased since the 1970s (Emanuel 2007).

By the end of the twenty-first century, storms are expected to be 2 to 11 percent stronger on average, meaning they are likely to become more destructive. In addition, models project that hurricanes will produce 20 percent more rainfall rates within the 100 km radius of the storm than they have been producing. This is a problem for coastal cities (Kossin, Olander, and Knapp 2013).

Hurricanes can result in both direct deaths (e.g., people who are killed during the storm due to wind or storm surge–induced drowning) and indirect deaths (e.g., CO_2 poisoning resulting from improper use of generators during power outages following a storm). The elderly are particularly vulnerable to both direct and indirect causes of death; hurricanes can cause a disruption of the power grids, and extreme weather following the storm, whether it be hot or cold, can pose a threat to vulnerable elderly (Gamble and Balbus 2016). The direct health impacts of weather-related events will be discussed further in chapter 5.

HARMFUL ALGAL BLOOMS

Intensive agriculture and the use of septic systems have increased the nutrient levels in water. Population density and intense lobbying on behalf of agriculture, pesticide companies, and developers have contributed to an exponential increase of nitrogen and phosphate levels in lakes and rivers. This provides food for bacteria and algae, which "bloom" (Barile et al. 2018). These algal blooms are caused by cyanobacteria that thrive in warmer temperatures (Falconer and Humpage 2005; Neilan et al. 2013). The increase in temperature has created a favorable environment for these bacteria and increased health problems for humans (Gobler et al. 2017; Falconer and Humpage 2005; Carmichael 2016). In the Pacific, exposure to algal blooms has been associated with symptoms of dementia, such as Alzheimer's disease (Cox et al. 2016). More common, however, is hepatotoxin exposure through drinking water, which can cause liver failure, and ultimately death (Falconer and Humpage 2005). Inhaling dust can also cause neurological problems like ALS (Lou Gehrig's disease) (Stommel, Field, and Caller 2013). The consistently warmer weather associated with global warming means that harmful algal blooms will become more frequent and affect waters farther from the equator (Gobler et al. 2017). Florida, known for its warm weather, has already seen an increase in harmful algal blooms during the summer months. It is unknown to what extent these blooms can affect people with underlying medical conditions.

DISASTERS DO NOT HIT EQUALLY

A theme in the coming chapters is that these disasters rarely impact all people in a society in the same ways. People with lower income are often unable to afford the protections that the more affluent can purchase. In Miami, Florida, for example, the cost of housing in slightly higher elevations is increasing (Bolstad 2017). Individuals who live in those areas are likely to be able to afford cars, plane tickets, hotel rooms, and insurance should a hurricane or flood hit the area where they live. There are many people who cannot afford those things.

In 2016, the National Institutes of Health and the Environmental Protection Agency partnered to produce research on how a changing climate can affect populations in different ways. They consolidated decades of findings to demonstrate that the impact of a changing climate can "vary by age and life stage" and that "social determinants of health interact to affect health risks" (Gamble and Balbus 2016). Further discussion of such social determinants of health, including the concept of syndemics, ecosyndemics, vulnerability, and expected loss, can be found in chapters 5 and 7.

DROUGHTS, HUMANITARIAN CONFLICT, AND REFUGEES

Research indicates that droughts, exacerbated by climate change, can lead to humanitarian conflicts (Châtel 2014; Kelley et al. 2015). More recently, researchers have found that droughts correlate with social disruption in many areas, suggesting a verifiable pattern (Almer, Laurent-Lucchetti, and Oechslin 2017). When basic needs are not met for large sections of a population, social conflicts spark. If a changing climate creates greater water scarcity and food shortages, people will fight to survive. Underlying social tensions will flare up.

The civil war in Syria, resulting in the refugee crisis in Europe, began with a drought that destabilized the country (Châtel 2014; Kelley et al. 2015). The NPR article "How Could a Drought Spark a Civil War" provides a synopsis of the complex history that began with an intense drought between 2006 and 2010 (National Public Radio 2013). "The four years of drought turned almost 60 percent of the nation into a desert . . . killing about 80% of the cattle by 2009" (2013). The article describes how subsistence, including agriculture and pastoralism, could no longer be sustained, forcing populations to migrate to cities to try to find work. Once in the cities, social class and religious affiliation affected their reception. Social conflicts began to erupt and became critical in the city of Dara'a after teenagers were arrested and beaten for writing pro–Arab Spring graffiti. These beatings sparked protests. In March 2011, security forces fired on the protesters. The uprising escalated. Hundreds of thousands have been killed (Rodgers et al. 2016). This humanitarian crisis crossed borders as 5.4 million people have fled Syria after chemical weapons were used against citizens ("Syria Emergency" 2018). This is only one example of how weather-related events can ignite or at least exacerbate social conflict. Like an oil spill or polluted air, humanitarian crises are rarely contained within geopolitical borders; they affect us all. Everyone, it seems, ought to be concerned with the increased frequency of droughts. Yet not everyone is convinced.

MISINFORMATION CAMPAIGNS

Though there is a wide range of quality scientific data from numerous environmental specialists, many citizens of the United States have become confused about the anthropogenic causes of a changing climate. This is largely the result of targeted misinformation campaigns, funded by a small number of wealthy individuals who have a vested interest in promoting an ongoing reliance on fossil fuels. The Koch brothers are well-known proponents (Clynes 2012; Getler 2015; Tankersley and Mooney 2016).

Scientific evidence is not always enough to convince policymakers or the public that action is required to protect public health. In 2013, *The Daily Show* ran clips of Fox News anchors expressing skepticism about climate change because of the exceptionally cold winter in 2014 (Stewart 2014). Stuart Varney, one host, followed up his tirade against the validity of climate change with the statement, "But, that is just my opinion" (Leiserowitz 2006). This was followed by a clip from *Fox and Friends* wherein they interviewed Donald Trump, then known only as a wealthy real estate developer and host of a reality television show. He called global warming a "hoax" because of the cold weather he was experiencing in New York in 2014. Even though neither Varney nor Trump cited valid scientific research, nor had the scientific credentials to make what they said more than their individual opinions, they were broadcast on a national news platform as if they were experts. The writers at *The Daily Show* used the commentators' lack of expertise on the topic of climate change as a source of humor, while also pointing out how the public was being misled.

In truth, 97 percent of qualified, highly trained environmental scientists understand both that the climate is changing more rapidly than it has in the past and that humans have contributed to this transformation (Anderegg et al. 2010). They also understand, as described above, that warming at the poles can create colder variations in lower latitudes. There is a small minority of climate scientists who are skeptical of the science, but most of the debate surrounds the specific details of *how much* the climate will warm over the next one hundred years (depending on different variables). Of note, over time, climate scientists have concluded that the planet is warming faster than they had previously realized (Mann et al. 2017). There are also long-standing methodological disagreements between those who do short-term weather analysis (meteorology) and those who model long-term climate changes (Mooney 2007).

Science is ultimately performed by humans within very real political-economic constraints and in a world of enormous complexity; as such, the pursuit of science is imperfect. Critical analysis from other experts (peer review) is essential and there is nearly always room for refining a knowledge base. While scientific debate is healthy, the "debate" over the existence and cause of global warming continues to be overstated in the media and in political forums for political and economic reasons (Dressler and Parson 2010). Since 2009, when *Citizens United* was decided, unlimited funds can be legally spent to influence legislators as they form policy (Wiist 2011; Lima and Galea 2018). This legislation has allowed for targeted misinformation campaigns and has caused confusion among lay populations who are already struggling to evaluate risks (Leiserowitz 2006). A 2012 Pew Research poll found that only 45 percent of the public thought "scientists believe the earth is getting warmer because of human activity" (Brulle 2013, 681). Francesca Pongiglione, an anthropologist who looks specifically at how people make decisions about climate change, argues that people have to (1) have knowledge, "in the form of basic scientific understanding and procedural knowledge," (2) recognize the risk (risk perception) to self or community, and (3) have a self-interest, either monetary or status driven (2012, 1). The targeted misinformation campaigns have worked to keep people from even basic knowledge, which in turn obscures a sense of risk. These structural factors fueling (dis)belief are part of the ecosocial conditions of the Elder Health Ecosyndemic.

SUMMARY

The **Elder Health Ecosyndemic** is rooted within the ecosocial. Since Mooney's documentation of the issues surrounding the climate change and hurricane debate, scientists have become even more certain that warming oceans are linked to stronger cyclonic storms such as hurricanes, but public uncertainty about the issue remains (2007).

There are macro-level economic processes that shape our current action and inaction toward climate turmoil. The impact happens at the micro level, affecting people on the ground. For anthropologists, climate change is not an abstract concept that "may . . . or may not" affect humanity in the far-off future; it is something we see impacting people now—the people with whom we are working, in communities around the globe, whether it be in the Sahara or the Arctic or in the United States (Crate and Nuttall 2009). It is happening before our eyes and we see people struggling to adapt. As such, it is personal. Anthropologists adhering to critical medical anthropology are charged with assisting those who have less power to exact political change. These are often the same people who will endure the most due to climate turmoil. We are watching as communities succumb to an increasingly warm climate that is taking away their livelihoods, their health, and their lives. Yet there is a discomfort with addressing the issues in the wider population. Further ideas on how to address these challenges are explored in chapter 10.

Chapter Four

Archaeology of Hurricanes

In 2015, I watched the Palm Beach County Historic Preservation Officer and Archaeologist, Chris Davenport, present archaeological findings from a site located along the banks of Lake Okeechobee, Florida. This site was discovered after a severe drought in 2006, when the South Florida Water Management District released water to prepare for hurricane season. This is done to ensure lower levels of water in case a hurricane hits the area. If the water levels are high, it is more likely that the water will overwhelm the Hoover Dike and flood the surrounding areas (Davenport and Mount 2007, 1). As a result of the coinciding drought and draining of the lake, parts of the lake bed were exposed for the first time since records had been kept, revealing new archaeological sites. These sites helped archaeologists better understand how people lived in the past and what their world was like (2007). One of the underlying purposes of archaeology is to re-create and understand past social and ecological conditions.

Across the globe, human history has been covered up by rising sea levels, though it is periodically revealed through short-term shifts in weather and underwater archaeology (Sassaman et al. 2017; Flemming et al. 2014). The short-term drought that revealed new archaeological sites in Florida was not indicative of a climate shift, at least not on its own. One of the most important tenets of climate change (and the source of much confusion among lay populations) is that although climate and weather are related phenomena, they are not the same thing. Climate is the long-term average conditions in a region over time. Weather is short-term temperature, rainfall, clouds, or wind on a day-to-day basis. Climate can only be determined by comparing averages over time.

For example, humans began to inhabit what is now known as the state of Florida approximately 13,000 years ago (Green 2016, 7). The landscape and *climate* the Paleoindians found were different from what is experienced today. "Florida was significantly cooler and drier . . . much of the water was frozen in glaciers farther north," which meant that sea levels were lower (2016, 7). Ultimately, Florida was twice the size it is today, and Lake Okeechobee did not yet exist.

Approximately 11,000 years ago, there was a slow climatic shift that brought with it warmer, wetter conditions and sea level rise (known as the Archaic period). The megafauna (mammoths and mastodons) began to go extinct, so the people who depended on them for food shifted their cultural traditions and adapted (Green 2016). With the rising sea, Lake Okeechobee and the Everglades formed, covering some of the evidence of human occupation, which was revealed in 2007 (Davenport and Mount 2007). The current sea level was reached and stabilized 2,500 to 5,000 years ago (Green 2016; Fagan 2013). That meant that, overall, the shift in climate happened over many generations.

The relatively slow climatic shift is important to note because many skeptics of climate change use the fact that there were climate shifts throughout history to downplay the change in climate we are witnessing now (see Lindzen 2009). It is important to note that earlier humans, in general, had a very different relationship with their environments than we do now. *Homo sapiens* have been on earth approximately three hundred thousand years (Bower 2017; Schlebusch et al. 2017). Intensive agriculture, which drove sedentary lifestyles, has only been a subsistence pattern for the past ten thousand years (Patin et al. 2009; Kelley et al. 2015). During the past one hundred years the settlement and subsistence patterns have shifted. As explained in chapter 8 on the built environment, most people now live in densely packed cities and are distanced from direct food production (Kramer, Khan, and Jahan 2011; Wisner and Uitto 2009).

For most of human history, nomadic lifestyles with semipermanent housing meant that as sea levels rose, people could relocate. As food sources died off during periods of historical climate change, people shifted and changed their diet and the tools used to obtain food (Munoz, Gajewski, and Peros 2010; Fagan 2008). If they did not, their maladaptive responses could have led to cultural extinction. Chapter 3 of Elert and Lemonick's book, *Global*

Weirdness, is titled "Our Ancestors Survived Climate Change. But It Wasn't Always Pretty" to briefly describe human responses to past climate change, while also explaining the underlying causes of those past shifts (Stein 1986). As Elert and Lemonick explain, "It's one thing for a small band of people to pack up camp and move a couple hundred miles to a better location if the climate changes. It's a very different thing to try to move a city like Cairo or New York or Shanghai because the sea level is rising" (2012, 19).

There is little evidence for agriculture in prehistoric Florida, but complex societies formed based on fishing, hunting, and foraging (Thompson and Pluckhahn 2010; White and Weinstein 2008). The ability of human populations to adapt to these climatic changes was at least partially rooted in the flexibility afforded by a hunting and gathering subsistence pattern.

ECOLOGICAL CONDITIONS OF THE PAST

Archaeologist Brian Fagan writes about sea level rise in *The Attacking Ocean: The Past, Present, and Future of Rising Sea Levels*, "One hundred and twenty meters and climbing: that's the amount of sea level rise since the end of the Ice Age some fifteen thousand years ago. Slowly, inexorably, the ascent continues in a warming world" (2013, 4). History, even of the climate, is informed by archaeology, which is the study of human remains and material culture with the goal of reconstructing how people lived in the past. Archaeologists do more than study the remains of buildings; they also look at flora and fauna so that they can understand how a population of people subsisted. Many archaeologists have training in paleolimnology (or work closely with geologists who have such training). Paleolimnology uses "cores" drilled from lake beds to reconstruct the paleoenvironment (Stein 1986). By examining the pollens and sediment in the cores, archaeologists can determine which plants were most common when a society lived at a particular locale. This information can be used to better understand the base of their subsistence pattern and specifics of their diets; it also gives clues as to what the environment might have been like. This is, in part, how scientists know that there was a shift from a dry climate in Florida to a wet one. Even more specifically, cores drilled from glaciers can tell scientists the composition of the atmosphere over time (Murray and Gaudet 2013). The climate record, established through ice and sediment cores (among other techniques), helps scientists reconstruct what was happening long before humans walked the earth; the record also tells us what kind of world humans lived in as they spread across the land. There are many other methods for determining local climate and diet from the past, including speleothem and data from caves, boreholes in the ground, and even isotopic analysis of human remains, which can give insights into diet and trade patterns ("Speleothem and Caves" 2017; "Borehole" 2017; Fiorenza et al. 2011).

ARCHAEOLOGY AND THE HISTORY OF CLIMATE IMPACT ON HUMANS

Humans have lived through extreme enviornmental flucuations in the past. For most of human history, we were migratory hunter-gatherers, who followed game animals or moved to find water and edible plants. Contrary to common conception, this subsistence pattern can be a stable one. Anthropological research on hunter-gatherer societies (the few that remain) shows that most calories are obtained through gathering, rather than hunting, and that there is far more leisure time than in farming or industrial societies (Lee 1968; Drapter 1975; Speth 1990; Ford, Grantham, and Whiting 2008). Food scarcity was less likely when there was ample territory in which to hunt and gather. The smaller population densities supported this subsistence pattern and also made adaption more rapid.

Our agricultural and industrial based civilizations were established during an unusually stable period in the environment (with some notable exceptions, such as the Little Ice Age (C. González et al. 2010; Fagan 2007; Elert and Lemonick 2012). This stable period has lasted for the past ten thousand years, during which time many societies adopted agricultural-based subsistence patterns. We now face an acceleration of climate-related events due to anthropogenic climate change. Unlike much of human history, our modern population densities and social arrangements, such as living in complex cities (especially in coastal areas), pose different challenges in responding to a continually disrupted environment. Without mitigating for increased storms through building codes, the scale of structural loss is greater and very costly to repair (Messner and Meyer 2006; O'Neill and Nicholson-Cole 2009; Kreimer, Arnold, and Carlin 2003; Kunreuther, Michel-Kerjan, and Ranger 2012).

Without public health interventions, such as educational campaigns, and risk communication, larger populations mean more people are at risk than ever before in human history. A higher number of elders who need special consideration means there is higher risk still; without prioritizing our elders through protective laws and regulations, they will continue to be expected to die (Fjord 2010).

Fagan provides a survey of the impact of climate on historical populations, large and small, in his 2004 book, *The Long Summer*. The most common cause of death during historical environmental changes was starvation due to prolonged drought or prolonged cold periods. The groups most vulnerable to climate changes were those dwelling in densely populated urban centers and relying on subsistence farming. Mobility and flexibility (i.e., being able to relocate to less affected areas) is what saved our predecessors from disaster on many occasions.

The causes of these prolonged droughts throughout human history were multifaceted. The global climate was impacted by factors such as a significant volcanic eruption anywhere in the world or by ice sheets melting, thereby introducing fresh water into the oceans, which interrupts the Gulf Stream cycle and familiar weather patterns. By comparing ice cores and tree rings, Fagan demonstrated how climate change influenced historical trends, showing repeatedly how civilizations large and small underwent complex changes or collapsed after historical climate events. He is careful to note that a person "cannot argue that climate drove history in a direct and causative way to the point of forcing major innovations or toppling entire civilizations. Nor, however, can one contend as many scholars once did that climate change is something that can be ignored" (Fagan 2004, xiv). He argued instead that smaller-scale, mobile societies (i.e., hunter-gatherer populations) were likely to be more resilient to major climate changes since they could easily adjust their location. This argument is supported by more recent archaeological work, documented in *Surviving Environmental Change: Answers from Archaeology*, edited by Jago Cooper and Payson Sheets (2012). In larger-scale societies, including predominantly sedentary ones such as our own, picking up and moving to more habitable climates is much more challenging.

It is beyond the scope of this book to outline all the complex factors that influence a changing global climate; however, a summary is laid out in the following pages. The most important facts related to the vulnerability of elders in a disrupted climate include: (1) oceans are warming, which fuels stronger hurricanes and cyclones (Trenberth 2007); (2) sea levels are rising due to melting ice caps and land ice, which means that storm surges are going to threaten greater areas along the coasts (Woodruff, Irish, and Camargo 2013; Romieu et al. 2010); (3) a warming climate will cause more heat waves, which is especially a problem if it coincides with power outages (frequently caused by storms) (Poumadere et al. 2005; Klinenberg 2013; Geggis and Chockey 2017); (4) a warmer climate is exacerbating underlying diseases, such as respiratory or cardiovascular diseases, and the spread of vector- and water-borne pathogens, while individuals with age-related cognitive diseases might have trouble making decisions that will keep them safe (Altizer et al. 2013; Semenza et al. 2012); and (5) eventually, water scarcity and food growth disruptions will also impact societies, as they have in Syria (Châtel 2014; Kelley et al. 2015). For each of these health-related expressions of climate change, vulnerable elders are at most risk.

A CASE STUDY

Jago Cooper, an archaeologist, researches pre-Columbian communities' responses to sudden environmental change, such as "floods, droughts, and wind shear created by relative sea level rise, precipitation change, and hurricane activity" on the Caribbean islands off the coast of Florida. In Cooper's chapter titled "Fail to Prepare, Then Prepare to Fail" in *Surviving Sudden Environmental Climate Change,* he focuses on the island of Cuba as a case study (2012). He points to mitigation strategies that include settlement location, subsistence strategies, and networks of community interactions.

The earliest archaeological evidence of human occupation in the Caribbean dates from approximately seven thousand years ago. At the time of this colonization, far more land was exposed, creating a far different coastline than we see today. Cuba, for example, has lost 27 percent of its landmass due to a five-meter sea level rise over the last six thousand years. Over this time, indigenous societies responded to these changes: "These earliest 'lithic' societies developed hunter-forager lifestyles in the Greater Antilles until around 4000 BP, when more complex lithic and shell artifacts and the more extensive colonization of other islands led to the 'archaic' phase of hunters, fishers, and foragers being defined" (Cooper 2012, 94).

A shift in subsistence patterns and social organization begins to emerge approximately 2,500 years ago. Evidence of ceramics and horticulture is found in the archaeological record at this time. Approximately 1,400 years ago (600 AD), more intensive agriculture was practiced in some communities, while others remained hunter-gatherers. There was trade between these two groups who had different subsistence patterns (Cooper 2012, 94).

Between AD 900 to 1492, there is archaeological evidence of "hierarchical societies and extensive networks of inter-island interaction" supporting a population of up to 1 million indigenous people across the Caribbean (Cooper 2012, 94). Both Florida and the pre-Columbian Caribbean areas are vulnerable to sea level rise, precipitation change, and hurricane activity, to which these people had to respond.

Sea Level Rise

Archaeological records tell us that "since the established colonization of the Caribbean, there has been at least a 5-meter rise in regional relative sea levels, which has radically changed the islandscape" (Cooper 2012, 96). Like modern-day Miami, the gradual sea level rise was punctuated by acute flooding events (*Science News* 2017, NBC6 2017).

Precipitation

Existing data indicate fluctuating regional precipitation rates over time, with a drier period beginning 10,500 BP, a wetter period beginning 7000 BP, and an intense drier period beginning 3,200 years ago (Higuera-Gundy et al. 1999: 159; Hodell et al. 1991; Nyberg et al. 2001).

Hurricanes

Cooper emphasizes that a hurricane event, while potentially deadly, is not the measure of the disaster; the true measure is how a community can recover. Hurricane Irma and Hurricane Maria, for example, were both dangerous hurricanes; however, the State of Florida had stronger building codes and better access to national resources than Puerto Rico, which was hit by both Hurricane Irma and Hurricane Maria, making the recovery efforts vastly different. The political landscape in which these storms occurred also changes the way that relief efforts and recovery are actualized. Like the present, Cooper argues that the recovery is what was most important for Cuban communities in the past.

Sedimentary cores from lagoons in Cuba and Puerto Rico show an identical hurricane history: heavy hurricane–intense periods from 4000 to 3600 BP, and then lower incidence of hurricanes until about 2600 BP (Peros et al. 2015; Donnelly and Woodruff 2007). A high number of hurricanes affected these islands between 2600 BP and 1000 BP (583 BCE through 1000 CE). There was a dip in hurricane activity, at least in these areas, between 1000 BP and 600 BP (1000 CE through 1400 CE). There was another drop in hurricane activity, which coincides with the Little Ice Age, from 600 BP to 300 BP (1400 CE to 1700 CE), when Atlantic Ocean temperatures were lower. Beginning in 1700, the hurricane activity increased sharply and has continued to do so within the last one hundred years.

Research Site: Los Buchillones, Cuba, from 1250 CE to 1492 CE

Settlement locations show that most pre-Columbian settlements in Cuba are located near caves, which could be used as temporary shelter during storms, and there was a preference for building communities on the leeward side of hills. "Paleoenvironmental evidence shows that the site was a Pre-Columbian residential settlement that straddled the coastline using stilted wooden structures over waterlogged environments" (Cooper 2012, 104). The stilts were made of local mahogany and lighter materials made up the living areas, thought to have thatched roofs. The stilts from these sites have remained in place for hundreds of years, with the upper living areas potentially rebuilt "from locally sourced materials" if damaged.

Today, most settlements are "located and founded by post-contact communities, predominately using European settlement planning traditions" (Larsen et al. 2001, 96). These communities, rather than being on the leeward side of hills, tend to be in river valleys, which are more vulnerable to flooding and storm surges. Many modern homes in Cuba are built of concrete, which can usually withstand hurricane winds. Roofing materials, however, are not locally sourced (like pre-Columbian homes) and can be expensive and time-consuming to replace.

The findings at this site may not be transferable to all communities that existed on the island during the same time, but some lessons may be relevant: diversification of food types from different environments, such as reefs, mangroves, and lowland agricultural and upland forest areas could have protected people from starvation; if one or two of these areas was damaged, in a hurricane for example, then they could supplement with food sources from other areas. Currently, Cuba has eight primary agricultural crops, which include inedible products, such as tobacco, or foods that are grown as cash crops and could not sustain a population alone, such as coffee and sugar cane. In 2017, Hurricane Irma damaged the eastern side of the island and "caused severe damage to livestock facilities, windmills, [and] crops" (ACN Cuban News Agency 2017). The preliminary report stated that around five thousand hectares (ha) of vegetables and fruits were damaged; of them 4,188 correspond to banana plantations. On this last product . . . everything in optimal state will be distributed to the population and the rest to animal consumption, and work is [being] done to recover those plantations. (ACN Cuban News Agency 2017)

The people of Cuba will need to rely heavily on international, imported foods for recovery.

Puerto Rico also suffered extreme loss of crops in 2017, due to Hurricane Irma and, more directly, Hurricane Maria. Hurricanes can decimate crops and transfers of supplies can be problematic, though not problematic enough to justify the delayed response after Hurricane Maria (Bump 2017; Robles and Ferre-Sadurni 2017).

We do not know the scale of deaths due to hurricanes in pre-Columbian Cuba, Puerto Rico, or Florida, but the settlement patterns and food acquisition strategies suggest a social structure resilient to these events. This is not to suggest their way of life was better or worse; it suggests that there were adaptions that included both an awareness of and preparation for hurricanes and potential floods.

As the waters ebbed and flowed, people could respond, perhaps, with more agility than my family and I could today, with our sedentary jobs, unmovable homes, and dependency on industrial agriculture and refrigerated supermarkets. The danger of hurricanes is not always in the direct hit, but in a community's ability to respond to the damage afterward.

"ELDERS" OF THE PALEOLITHIC

While bioarchaeologists have provided preliminary estimates, it is difficult to specifically judge the life expectancies during the Paleolithic. The Paleolithic environment likely posed similar challenges to elders as they face today (such as heat stress); however, life expectancy appears to be lower in the past than it is now. Bioarchaeological research from pre-Columbian human remains in four different Florida sites showed an average age of death in their early twenties (ages 21.3, 22.5, 23.0, and 23.2) (Larsen et al. 2001). The mean age overall is higher in the post-contact site (aged 29.8 at time of death), but this may be due to lower birthrates after contact and therefore fewer children showing up in the archaeological record to balance the averages (Larsen et al. 2001, 96). The proportion of adults living beyond the age of 45 in the pre-Columbian samples was sometimes very small, making up less than 1 percent (.6%; n=2) of the 316 individuals at one site. The largest proportion of people over 40 was 12.5 percent (n=21) of 168 individuals at another pre-Columbian site. People over the age of 45 made up 23.7 percent (27/114) of the post-contact mission population. It is difficult to postulate exactly how much of an effect these historical weather-related events might have had on older individuals based on these data alone.

Florida is now densely populated, with approximately 18,801,000 residents as of 2010. Of these, 44 percent are over the age of 45 ("Florida Population by Age Group" 2016). Making the claim that "climate changes happened in the past, so we will be fine now" fails to consider (1) that the speed at which the climate is changing is faster than in the past; (2) the built environments in which we live are different, often culturally informed; and (3) the social makeup of our societies is different. Current climatic shifts and the resulting increase in weather-related disasters are putting more people at risk than in the past. The extent to which we work to reduce the potential suffering and death is a measure of our values.

SUMMARY

We face a climatic shift that is unlike the gradual changes experienced by the Paleoindians. Our climate is warming faster. The sea levels are rising faster, too. At the same time, our population is far denser. We can summarize vast amounts of archaeological and climatological findings to state that though humans have long responded to climate-related changes and disasters, our current social structures make it more difficult to quickly adapt to the current and predicted climate turmoil. Elders are particularly vulnerable to these changes. Now that we are sedentary and have built up dwellings along coasts, we have a lot at risk: lives, especially the lives of elders and children, as well as infrastructure. However, we have the knowledge and technology to address these deaths. Not to do so is a choice we make as a society because it is expensive and challenging.

Chapter Five

Aging Theory

The electricity in my middle-class neighborhood was restored a week after Hurricane Irma hit. Though my in-laws lived only a mile away (in an adjacent neighborhood), their power remained out for another week. Cousins who lived in more rural areas also had prolonged power outages. All of us, however, also had a swimming pool, a car, access to a generator, fuel, and supplies. Another part of town, Dunbar, which was less affluent and had less access to disaster supplies (let alone swimming pools), also remained without power. Disasters happen within a historical and ecosocial context. The results can play out differently across socioeconomic class systems.

THE HISTORICAL AND ECOSOCIAL CONTEXT OF DUNBAR, LEE COUNTY, FLORIDA

In 1962, the City of Fort Myers purchased land in a historically black neighborhood called Dunbar. This land was not used for construction or for a park, but rather, it was used as a site to dump waste from a water treatment plant (Borns 2017). Dunbar was the site of the only all-black school in southwest Florida. Students were bused in from an hour away to attend the segregated school (Rosenberg 2014). Though the *Brown v. Board of Education* ruling mandated the desegregation of schools in 1954, it was a full decade later, 1964, when Lee County, Florida, was forced to address its lack of integration (Smith 2014). While the NAACP was representing twenty students against Lee County for refusing to desegregate the schools, a bust of Robert E. Lee was erected in the center of downtown Fort Myers in 1966 (Dorsey 2017;

Parks 2017; Smith 2014). Desegregation was stalled until 1969, when schools were forced to reorganize. It took until 1999 for the high schools to be granted "unitary status," meaning they met the standard of desegregation (Smith 2014). As of 2014, Dunbar High remains a minority majority school (50 percent of the students are black, 27 percent Hispanic, 19 percent white non-Hispanic) (Rosenberg 2014). Those who graduated from the first integrated schools are now in their sixties as of 2018. This is not ancient history.

The toxic sludge buried in Dunbar land remains a microcosm of institutionalized racism that permeates much of the United States: the sludge, buried in the segregated area of the county, has been releasing unsafe levels of arsenic into the soil and water for almost sixty years (Borns 2017). Though the unsafe levels of arsenic were discovered in Dunbar's water in 2008, the residents were not notified, no signs were posted, no fences prevented children from playing in that area (Borns 2017; Nemec 2008). It is unknown how, if at all, this sludge dump has affected the community's health. Several residents wonder if the multiple cases of cancers in their families are related. They want to know but are not sure who to ask. To access cancer registries, a person must have special permissions.

David Hodges, an investigative reporter at NBC2 News, did a segment before Hurricane Irma, exploring how flooding resulting from Hurricane Irma might affect the areas surrounding the toxic sludge dump (Hodges 2017a). Hodges requested comment from the Florida Department of Environmental Protection (DEP) and a Florida Gulf Coast University (FGCU) environmental studies professor, Dr. L. Donald Duke. The DEP said that site visits were done before the hurricane to document all site conditions. Duke said that the risks of the Dunbar site caused minimal concern and named many other sites that were more dangerous.

For most people, though, toxic sludge is just one of the many risks faced after a hurricane. Transportation to stores was limited and so were funds to purchase these things. Investing in a disaster kit, something to be saved for later emergency, requires having money to invest in food and supplies that are not needed immediately. Many people do not have such excess funds: they live paycheck to paycheck, sometimes meal to meal. The Elder Health Ecosyndemic explains how the social conditions, including the historical devaluing of the lives of black people in the United States, can amplify health conditions that might exist for all elders. When this interacts with the ecosocial effects of a changing climate, vulnerability is increased.

CRITICAL MEDICAL ANTHROPOLOGY

Socioeconomic status (including age, race, and economic standing) influences a person's susceptibility to disease and vulnerability to disaster. Some political, social, and economic processes exacerbate (or even cause) greater vulnerability to disease and disaster. Critical medical anthropology (CMA) is a highly self-reflective theoretical orientation to anthropological work that draws attention to how social processes (such as age, race, class, and ethnicity) and the biology behind diseases are tightly intertwined.

A critical medical anthropology paradigm is presented in the book *Unhealthy Health Policy: A Critical Anthropological Examination*. Arachu Castro and Merrill Singer, the book's editors, clearly outline the distinctive aspects of critical medical anthropology:

> The CMA perspective (1) recognizes that health itself is a profoundly political issue, one that often is contentious if not explosive; (2) is cognizant and critical of the colonial heritage of anthropology and the tendency of conventional medical anthropology to serve as a "handmaiden of biomedicine"; (3) balances concern for unbiased social science with an awareness of the sociohistoric origin and political nature of all scientific knowledge; (4) acknowledges the fundamental importance of class, racial and sexual inequity in determining the distribution of health, disease, living and working conditions, and health care; (5) defines power as a fundamental variable in health-related research, policy, and programming; (6) avoids the artificial separation of local settings and micropopulations from their wider political-economic contexts; (7) asserts that its mission is emancipatory: it aims not simply to understand but also to change culturally inappropriate, oppressive, and exploitative patterns in the health arena and beyond; and (8) sees commitment to change as fundamental to the discipline. (Castro and Singer 2004, xiv)

Locating the study of health policy within critical medical anthropology clarifies health-related social situations because it "emphasizes the importance of political and economic forces, including the exercise of power, in shaping health, disease, illness experience, and health care" (Castro and Singer 2004, xiv). Critical medical anthropology considers some of the structural barriers that might prevent people from adopting risk reducing behaviors; thus, a critical medical anthropologist would ask why might a person fail to compile a disaster kit or evacuate for a hurricane, even if they are armed with information and believe themselves to be at risk? Poverty, for example, can be a barrier for some families who do not have money to spend on stockpiling canned goods or investing in a generator. Not all families have access to transportation. Individuals suffering from a temporary or chronic illness might be physically unable to easily evacuate. Being an ethnic minority may be a factor in receiving storm preparedness information or, as seen in Hurricane Katrina, poor sections of cities may suffer delays in getting rescue and emergency services. Others might not have a social network to assist them in an emergency. Critical medical anthropology considers the many social, economic, and political factors that can influence a person's willingness and ability to respond to a public health emergency in the way that public health professionals wish.

SOCIAL CONSTRUCTION OF AGING, HEALTH, AND ILLNESS

While aging is a biological factor, the meanings and behaviors attached to specific ages are socially constructed (Hendricks and Hendricks 1976). How we think about age can influence a person's social role and how they are valued in society. The value of elders in a society can impact whether or not they are fully considered in disaster planning at local and national levels.

Time, Age, and the Life Course

Humans tend to stratify themselves by age. Anthropologist Christine Fry writes, "Humans have 'domesticated time' by making it a subject of cultural interpretation" (2007, 7). Cultural interpretation results in a variation of how "age" is defined and measured across different societies (Hendricks and Hendricks 1976; Fry 2007). Not all societies measure age against the number of rotations the earth has made around the sun since they were born; this measure (incorporated into the Gregorian calendar) is a relatively recent invention (Fry 2002). More general markers, such as changing seasons, might be used as an indicator for change over time. Another way to conceptualize age is to categorize people into generations (or generational life courses), life stages (staged life courses), or age-classed life courses. In modern Western societies, age—measured from the time of birth—has become an important biomarker that is codified in legal and medical documents and is assumed to correlate with certain stages in human development, denoting "citizenship" and legal status as an "adult."

Chronological age (in most modern, Western societies) is divided into a "tripartite" life course, which divides citizenship into three stages: (1) childhood, (2) adult citizenship, and (3) postadulthood or old age (Fry 2007; Cattell and Albert 2009). Conceptions about age-specific roles and responsibilities can vary across societies; for example, while people are considered to have the capacity to consume alcoholic beverages in Germany at the age of sixteen, people in the United States must wait until twenty-one to gain legal sanction for drinking (at least in public). In modern times, adulthood is a period when a person is capable of "full citizenship," as demonstrated by roles taken in family relations and work (or the provision of goods) (Estroff 1993). As a result, when one reaches "postadult" status, a person often relinquishes responsibilities, such as working full-time, as had Joe and Betsy Dunmore in their retirement. Thus, there are different social roles and responsibilities (or lack thereof) associated with different stages of the human life course. In a capitalist society, it is possible to devalue those who are no longer generating capital for the system. In some cases, especially when a person has a disability that renders them unable to care for themselves, they may lose their adult status legally and socially (Estroff 1993). Robert Murphy, an anthropologist who was struck with a debilitating illness at the height of his career, wrote about this loss of social status in his work *The Body Silent* (1987). Murphy explains the expectation of reciprocity in social relationships and how disability can alter the balance: "Over-dependency and non-reciprocity are considered childish traits, and adults who have them—even if it is not their fault—suffer from a reduction of status" (Murphy 1987, 201). Murphy describes the resulting social shift within his family: "During the years of my illness, I have become transformed from active father and husband, the source of help and support for Yolanda and the children, to passive recipient of services" (Murphy 1987, 212). There are several diseases that are associated with older age that can cause such disabilities. More recently, Dr. Richard Taylor, trained as a psychologist, used voice recognition software to document the diagnosis and progression of his Alzheimer's disease (Taylor 2007). Like Murphy, Taylor describes a sense of loss: his identity as an academic, and eventually, the loss of his status as an independent adult.

NORMAL AGING AND AGING-RELATED DISEASES

According to critical medical anthropology, understanding dementia within a historical context is vital to illustrating how it has been socially constructed. Here I use the concept of dementia as an aging-related disease to explore the concepts of disease and illness, and normal versus pathological aging. Finally, I discuss other aging-related diseases, how they are conceptualized, and how people with such diseases can become more vulnerable during disasters.

Older age is the strongest correlate and risk factor for Alzheimer's disease and related dementias; the most common form appears after the age of sixty (Bludau 2010). An anthropologist who adheres to a critical medical anthropology perspective, Bludau deconstructs the sociohistoric origins of the scientific knowledge about a disease, in this case, Alzheimer's disease. Anthropologists consider who decides and how decisions are made about defining and measuring diseases. The definitions and designations are linked with policy and power; those who define and relegate Alzheimer's disease into different funding streams determine who and what aspects of the disease are funded (Christensen 2012; Lock 2013). Whether the person with the disease or the person who provides care for them is of interest can determine how disease research is funded (or not funded). In this way, the framing of disease is largely in the hands of health policymakers and those who are able to influence the formulators of social policy (Christensen 2012; Kaufman 1988, 2006; Lock 2013). In the United States, funding is heavily skewed toward biomedical and high-tech-oriented solutions over other forms of treatment (such as social work contact or hospice interventions) that might reduce stress for both the person suffering with an affliction and their caregivers.

Arguments that posit dementia as a "normal" part of aging have been pitted against those that conceptualize it as a disease distinct from the aging process. These debates provide context in which dementia and Alzheimer's disease, specifically, began to be medicalized. The naming of the disease (and the identification of the organic structures associated with its signs and symptoms) created a jumping-off point from which the medical field could begin to measure and diagnose the illness (Kaufman 1988). According to anthropologist Sharon Kaufman, historically, people assumed that senility was a normal (and therefore inevitable) part of growing old, until the idea came under scrutiny in the late 1880s. A physician, I. L. Nascher, began arguing that memory loss was not, in fact, a normal part of aging (Kaufman 2006). People who experienced senility, he said, had a disease. The debate over whether the "softening of the brain" was a normal part of aging and whether aging itself was a pathological or a chronic illness, continued through the 1930s, and the "aging as a disease" paradigm continued to be taught in medical schools (Kaufman 2006, 26).

In many ways, the debate continues to this day (Blumenthal 2003; Lock 2013). In the modern era, even with the use of scientific measurement, the boundaries between normal aging and disease remain blurred (Lock 2013). In 2013, medical anthropologist Margaret Lock documented how scientists struggled to understand the root causes of Alzheimer's disease, which have yet to be resolved. As Kaufman points out, "the idea of age-related disease muddies the waters" about whether there is a difference between "normal aging" and "aging as disease" (2006, 26). The case of arteriosclerosis is a good example of this, since it is normal to have age-related hardening of the arteries "until it progresses to a point at which they lead to diseases, such as heart attacks" (Blumenthal 1993, 1272—as quoted in Kaufman 2006). Once a person has a heart attack, the hardened arteries are no longer "normal"— they are considered "pathological." Similarly, forgetfulness is now considered to be a normal part of aging, until it reaches a point when a person can no longer complete their activities of daily living (ADL) (Teunisse and Derix 1997). Thus, while aging is associated with several normal conditions, once they progress to a certain (socially and medically defined) point they become age-related diseases. In the decades since the identification and naming of Alzheimer's disease, the debate over where to draw the lines has continued.

In one respect, "naming a disorder can bring order out of chaos" and offers the possibility of resolution (Womack 2010, 84). This allows, for example, a concerned spouse to "see" the disease in order to fulfill a general psychological need to define and order a chaotic experience and provides clear expectations for the future, which, though bleak, are more secure than the unknown (Gubrium 1986; Herskovits 1995; Whitehouse et al. 2005). Once named, a disease is defined by its signs and symptoms. The severity of the signs and symptoms can then be measured, and a search begun for causes and ways to reduce them.

Diagnosis also brings with it legitimacy (Kleinman 1980). "[W]hatever the patient's experience of pain, disability, or illness might be," affirms Solimeo, "this experience must be validated by a health care practitioner in order for a patient to legitimately be sick" (Solimeo 2009, 9). Establishing the legitimacy of an illness can result in desired social acceptability as well as resources for the suffering person. For instance, in Florida, dementia must be diagnosed by a medical professional in order to obtain financial support for medical and social services (Christensen 2012). The medical professional evaluates the physical signs and symptoms with a number of tests and measurements. The severity of the cognitive impairments is ranked to determine the types and amounts of formal support that can be offered. This might all seem like a straightforward medical procedure. Yet anthropologists emphasize that the process of naming and defining a disease is culturally driven. As explained by Whitehouse et al.:

> Although AD [Alzheimer's disease] and other subdiagnoses are considered discrete categories for which specific therapies are sought, in actual fact, the boundaries that might delineate the various dementias, and distinguish between normal and abnormal cognitive functioning, are unclear and are constantly debated within the medical professions. (2005, 321)

Beyond biomedical explanations, alternative explanatory models might be employed by patients to cope with an unfamiliar disease; many of these have been documented by medical anthropologists (Kaufman 2006; Ikels 2002). For example, Cohen found that, in India, the locus of Alzheimer's disease is believed to lie in "a bad family" (read broken, scattered, inattentive, and neglectful family) (Cohen 1998). People who lived with intact, "good" families, it was assumed, did not become senile. In another anthropological study, Annette Leibing found that many families thought that the true cause of Alzheimer's disease was a "hard life" that the afflicted person could no longer process (Cohen 1998). Ikels, in a study in Guangzhou, China, illustrated that while people might display the same physiological and behavioral features of dementia, their experience of the disease is very different from those with dementia in the United States (Kaufman 2006; Ikels 2002). These differences lie within the social makeup of the societies and in "meaning attributed to these changes and in the caregiving arrangements" (Hashmi 2009, 209).

Alzheimer's type dementia is only one type of disease associated with older age that is caught between biology and cultural definition. As previously mentioned, up until the 1930s, medical schools taught that the process of growing older or aging was a type of disease (Gamble et al. 2013). Today, gerontologists recognize that a person over the age of sixty is not automatically frail or vulnerable; many people over the age of sixty, like Betsy, remain physically and mentally active (Mayhorn 2005). Biomedicine now distinguishes between normal aging and age-related pathology. For example, while it is normal for there to be a small degree of sensory decline as one ages, it is not considered normal for it to impair a person's ability to function or perform activities of daily living (Katz et al. 1970; Lawton and Brody

1969). When a person's ability to function is impaired, decline is considered pathological, in biomedical terms.

For example, to have some loss of eyesight as one ages is normal. Presbyopia, a slow loss of ability to see close objects or small print, does not alarm one's doctor because this is accepted as a normal part of the aging process (Truscott and Zhu 2010). While inconvenient, a person with presbyopia can usually still read a newspaper's small print by holding it at arm's length. A degree of hearing loss is also categorized as a normal part of aging. Minor hearing loss does not usually impair a person's ability to care for themselves and, like presbyopia, does not overly concern medical professionals. Tools, such as glasses or hearing aids, can reduce the inconvenience of these aging-related changes (Gamble et al. 2013). In the case of disaster planning and response, these minor impairments have the potential to change how a person responds in a disaster: these sensory changes might impact an older person's ability to see, hear, and ultimately understand disaster warning messages (Mayhorn 2005).

In addition to sensory changes, the body's ability to regulate internal temperature also declines, making older individuals more susceptible to hyperthermia (heatstroke) or hypothermia (a dangerous drop in core body temperature) (Hutton 2008; Van Someren 2007). This is problematic during extreme weather events or after a disaster should power be lost, causing household environmental controls such as air-conditioning or central heat to not function. As recently as 2017, eleven residents at a Florida skilled nursing facility died of complications from excessive heat after Hurricane Irma caused power outages (Huriash 2017; Spencer, Kay, and Reynolds 2017).

Other diseases correlated with older age affect the cardiorespiratory and metabolic systems. The risk of acquiring a chronic disease such as diabetes, Alzheimer's disease, or atherosclerosis (pathological hardening of the arteries) increases as one ages. Cardiovascular disease is a major cause of death worldwide and the most common cause of death in the United Sates ("Cardiovascular Diseases" 2017). These age-related diseases can (1) be exacerbated by environmental factors and (2) increase a person's vulnerability when environmental hazards, such as hurricanes and flooding, strike.

SUMMARY

The way age is measured and defined in Western societies is not universal. How age and social roles are defined is important because that can change

the ways in which laws and policies are written and influence what is prioritized. Thinking carefully about how age, disease, and disability can potentially help medical practitioners and lawmakers reduce structural vulnerabilities.
Older age is correlated with higher incidences of diseases and disabilities,
some temporary, some chronic. There is an ongoing debate over which conditions are a part of normal aging and which are part of a disease process. I
refer to these conditions broadly as "age-related diseases." Understanding the
cultural, social, ecological, and economic contexts in which these age-related
disease processes operate can better prepare nurses, doctors, public health
professionals, social workers, emergency managers, and urban planners to
respond to (and reduce) vulnerabilities (see chapter 8). In the next chapter, I
explore how climate change can exacerbate age-related diseases and, in turn,
make people more vulnerable to extreme weather events.

Chapter Six

Aging, Disability, and Disasters

Mili Bonillia flew to Puerto Rico a month after Hurricane Maria hit the island. She came because her father, Jose, was having trouble breathing (Jorgensen 2017). He was diagnosed with pneumonia, something that under normal circumstances could be easily treated. When the hospital ran out of oxygen and then lost power, the respirator became useless. Jose was dead within a week (Barbaro 2018).

In 2017, Puerto Rico was first impacted by Hurricane Irma, then directly hit by Hurricane Maria. Hurricane Maria was like a 50-mile tornado crossing the island, meaning that the entire area was affected (Resnick and Barclay 2017). Short of leaving by plane, there was nowhere to evacuate to. Those who went to shelters were unable to even reach hospitals if they needed to after the storm (Nedelman 2017). Nursing homes and hospitals were without power for months and the weather was hot (Feere-Sadurni, Robles, and Alvarez 2017). The official death toll attributed to Hurricane Maria stood at sixty-five (Robles 2017). People like Jose, who would, under normal circumstances, survive his illness, were not being counted in the official death toll. Yet the excess deaths were more than 50 percent from the previous year. Electricity was still not fully restored to the island four months after Hurricane Maria.

In 2016, the Puerto Rico census reported that approximately 5 percent of the population is under five years old; nearly 19 percent is over sixty-five. Of those who are *under* the age of sixty-five, 15 percent have a disability ("US Census Quick Facts Puerto Rico" 2016).

DEMOGRAPHICS

The Elder Health Ecosyndemic includes social conditions of an increasing older population. The aging population in the United States is growing, as are the number of people with age-related illnesses who are more vulnerable to hurricanes and the conditions that follow them.

Betsy and Joe Dunmore's experiences during the 2004 hurricanes, described in chapter 1, were unique in some ways; in other ways, their experiences demonstrate conditions faced by a growing number of individuals in the United States. In 2011, the first American baby boomers reached the age of sixty-five, the official retirement age. According to the AARP, since 2011 approximately eight thousand people turned sixty-five every day (Love 2010). By 2030, people over the age of sixty-five will make up approximately 20 percent of the US population (Uhlenberg 2013).

The United States is not alone in the increase in aging populations; most developed countries, Western Europe and Japan, for example, are also experiencing a decline in fertility and an increase in life expectancy (Muramatsu and Akiyama 2011). In fact, countries such as Spain and Japan are aging much more rapidly than the United States. Other countries are also experiencing a decrease in birth rates; China's older (over sixty-five population) nearly doubled between 1950 and 2014 and is expected to reach 30 percent of the total population by 2060 (Uhlenberg 2013, 14). These demographics do not require alarm, though China's former one-child policy and lack of pensions could potentially skew its ability to respond to the exceptionally rapid rate of growth of the aging population (Kaufman 2006, 25).

Though there are many positive aspects of an aging society, it is nonetheless important to explore the connection between health and aging overall, especially within the context of environmental and climate changes. Health and illness exist on a continuum with "normal" age-associated changes on the one hand and "pathological" conditions on the other (see table 6.1). The greatest risk factor for many chronic diseases, such as cardiovascular disease and Alzheimer's disease, is advanced age. Many of the precursors for these diseases are a normal part of aging. For example, it is normal for the arteries to accumulate some fatty buildup and lose elasticity over time; however, blockages of the arteries are considered pathogenic and are labeled as a disease (Bludau 2010). Pathogenic expression can be a combination of genetic predisposition and lifestyle (for example, smoking or eating a high-fat diet), diabetes, and is associated with chronic infections of herpes simplex virus type 1 (HSV-1), cytomegalovirus (CMV), and chlamydia pneumoniae (Nabipour et al. 2006).

Some difficulty retaining or recalling memories is a normal part of aging; however, extreme memory loss and behavioral changes are indicative of a disease that causes dementia (such as Alzheimer's disease or vascular dementia). Biomedically, these diseases are diagnosed through a combination of cognitive tests such as the Mini Mental Status Examination (MMSE) and magnetic resonance imaging (MRI) (Folstein, Folstein and McHugh 1975; Solomon et al. 1998). As explained in chapter 1, historically, senility (or severe memory loss) was a normal part of growing old. In the 1800s doctors began to argue that memory loss was not a normal part of the aging process (Kaufman 2006, 25). Today, gerontologists recognize that while the speed of memory recall might slow as one ages, severe memory loss and dementia are not a normal part of aging.

In addition, normal aging brings with it a slowing of the metabolism, which in turn can trigger changes in body fat composition. In extreme cases, this can trigger diabetes. Recently, diabetes and metabolic changes have been linked with Alzheimer's disease (Correia et al. 2012; Shah, Desilva, and Abbruscato 2012). People frequently have more than one of these chronic diseases at a time; in other words, there is a "highly prevalent aging-dependent phenomenon of multiple coexisting diseases" called comorbidities (Solomon 1999, 143). As discussed in chapter 5, syndemics are comorbidities that are not merely coexistent but are interactive, leading to enhanced disease burden (Singer and Clair 2003). Moreover, syndemic research offers us an

Table 6.1.   Normal Aging versus Pathological Disease

Normal Aging	Disease or Pathology
Some hardening of the arteries	Heart disease Blockage of arteries to the point that blood cannot reach critical areas, such as the heart, brain, or lungs
Cellular changes to skin and vital organs	Malignant neoplasms (cancer)
Slower metabolism	Diabetes mellitus (type II diabetes) Inability to secrete insulin
Loss of flexibility and decrease in joint tissue	Osteoarthritis
Slower recall and less retention	Alzheimer's disease Forgetting names of familiar people; becoming lost in familiar places

important anthropological perspective into the synergistic interactions between interacting comorbidities and the health effects of social conditions.

AGE-RELATED DISEASES AND DISABILITY

Disability can be defined as "an impairment in body functioning, limitations in activities, and restrictions in participation" (Binstock and George 2011, 77). Diseases that cause disability increase with older age. In the United States, approximately 35.2 percent of the population aged sixty-five and older has a disability of some kind (Kraus 2018, 8). (The number of people over sixty-five with a disability jumps to nearly 40 percent of the population in many of the American southern states.) Some of these impairments can restrict a person's abilities to fully participate in society and can require assistance to accomplish activities of daily living (ADLs), such as the ability to dress and feed oneself (Katz 1963). As the above table indicates, normal aging, as well as what is considered a "disease," can exist on a continuum of "expected" to "less expected" and possibly "deadly" (Kaufman 2006).

There are several illnesses that are not a normal part of aging and are labeled as a disease. Many of these illnesses are associated with older age. For example, an estimated 5.5 million Americans of all ages have Alzheimer's disease in 2017. Of these, 5.3 million are age sixty-five and older, and 200,000 individuals under age sixty-five have younger-onset Alzheimer's (Alzheimer's Association 2017, 18).

FRAIL ELDERLY

Not all people over the age of sixty-five have a disease or are disabled. Many are highly active. However, some older individuals might be categorized as "frail," and therefore especially vulnerable during a disaster. Geriatricians began to recognize frailty as a clinically recognizable syndrome among elders in the 1990s (Fulop et al. 2010; Mhaoláin et al. 2012). Fernandez and colleagues define frail elderly as "individuals aged 65 and older with physical, cognitive, social, psychological, and/or economic circumstances that will likely limit their ability to perform, or have performed for them, one or more Activities of Daily Living (ADLs) in Instrumental Activities" (Fernandez et al. 2002, 71).

Frailty, though difficult to measure clinically, is recognized as an overall decline in function or "reserve" (Funlop et al. 2010). Fulop et al. explain that "frailty is a nonspecific state of vulnerability, which reflects multisystem physiological changes. The set of changes underlying frailty do not always achieve disease status, so some people, usually very elderly, are frail without a specific diagnosed life-threatening illness" (2010, 547). Most "frail elderly" are among the "oldest old." Social scientists have begun to distinguish between the young-old (sixty-five) and the oldest old (eighty-five and older) (Fernandez et al. 2002). Frailty, however, at any age, can make a person more likely to become disabled, sustain environmental-related injury, and be put at higher risk for accelerated cognitive and physical decline than the general population.

AGING AND DISABILITY DURING HURRICANES

People over the age of sixty bore a disproportionate burden during Hurricane Katrina and Hurricane Sandy, which demonstrates the vulnerability of older populations to hurricanes. It can be more difficult for people with age-related diseases or disabilities to respond to disasters. Some of the increased risk to older populations can be explained by social structures, and to an extent, can be mitigated by social networks. Below, I give examples of how age, underlying illness, environmental conditions, and social structures can interact during a hurricane.

Hurricane Katrina

The Robin family, described in Ken Wells's book *The Good Pirates of the Forgotten Bayous*, demonstrates the difficulty of evacuating someone with Alzheimer's disease, especially if the caregiver had medical conditions as well (2008). It also describes key features of coastal living. Wells interviewed survivors of Hurricane Katrina in St. Bernard Parish. He explains that many residents of the area were suffering from evacuation fatigue from hurricanes that had hit but ultimately caused very little damage: "Many who have dutifully heeded past warnings and made the slow, expensive, frustrating, traffic-snarled evacuation to points north [had] grown weary of the voyage. A widespread skepticism of the accuracy of hurricane forecasting [had] set in" (Wells 2008, 29).

One of the families Wells describes is the Robin family: a family with a long history of fishing in the Louisiana bayous. Before Hurricane Katrina hit, Susan Robin, the matriarch, was recovering from back surgery while caring for her children and her father who was diagnosed with early-stage Alzheimer's disease. Susan's back injury made it difficult to evacuate the family upon Hurricane Katrina's approach. Her father's condition also played an important part in their decision to shelter in place:

> Sidney T., in his day, had been something of swamp lion—a carpenter by vocation but a man who, like many in these parts, supplemented the family larder as a gifted hunter and trapper. His progressive Alzheimer's has required him to be under constant medical care. All of his doctors (and hers) are in St. Bernard Parish. Evacuation, even for a few days, would have required her to find reliable backup care in whatever place they chose to dodge the storm. It seemed not just a hassle, but risky as well. (Wells 2008, 29)

Ricky Robin, the patriarch, was manning his boat as he had during past storms, while the family sheltered at home. When the levees broke, Susan noted the rising water in the streets and evacuated her family in a van. Wells narrates the evacuation:

> Susan bulls her way into the van, cranks it up, backs out, makes a U-turn, and steers it into position, with the loading doors as close to the front of the house as she can manage. She rushes back in to help secure her dad. Short of being physically carried out, her father simply can't be hurried . . . so between them all they essentially drag Sidney T. to the van and get him cinched in with a seatbelt in the back seat. . . . In that time, the water has already risen about another foot—and it is beginning to enter the house. (Wells 2008, 29)

The only place safe from the storm surge and the onslaught from the broken levee was up on the levee walls themselves, which is where the family maneuvered their van. From this vantage point, they see people being swept from their homes. It is here that the family spent the night.

Wells also describes the plight of Martine, ninety years old, who lived in the same area near the Violet canal with her seventy-one-year-old disabled son. Wells notes that Martine was able-bodied, gardening, doing chores, cooking traditional dishes, and looking after her son who had sustained a brain injury in a car accident. She had successfully survived Hurricane Betsy in 1965, partly because her home was on higher ground than some of the surrounding areas. Her previous success, and her concern about her son who did not fare well with changes to his environment, factored into her decision to shelter at home during Katrina. Her son, though gentle, refused to leave the home.

When Katrina hit, and the levees broke, Martine and her son evacuated their flooded home in a relative's canoe. When they left, they were without supplies. They found their way to the top of the levee and camped for the night with the Robin family. Later, Ricky Robin would reunite with his family and contribute to the rescue efforts. He would also have one of the first views of St. Rita's nursing home, which will be discussed further in chapter 9, on long-term care and disasters.

Post-Katrina Hyperthermia

Elderly populations are more vulnerable to heat-related illnesses. Heat can exacerbate other chronic conditions, such as respiratory illnesses or cardio-vascular disease. Unlike Hurricane Sandy, temperatures after Hurricane Katrina in 2005 were high; in the New Orleans area, the temperature was recorded to be 90°F (32°C) in the week following the storm ("New Orleans, LA, Week of August 28, 2005" 2005). While not considered a heat wave, high temperatures can cause sunstroke, heat cramps, and heat exhaustion with prolonged exposure and/or prolonged physical activity ("Heatwave: A Major Summer Killer"). (The World Meteorological Organization's definition for "heat wave" is when the daily maximum temperature for more than five consecutive days exceeds the average maximum temperature by 5°C, or 9°F, the normal period being 1961–1990). Under normal circumstances, these temperatures rarely are a threat to public health; however, in the days following Hurricane Katrina, most of New Orleans had lost power. Loss of power extended even to hospitals and nursing homes where staff and patients (not to mention people stranded in their homes) were exposed to prolonged high temperatures without air-conditioning. The impact of these temperatures can be measured in human life. Brunkard, Namulanda, and Ratard reported that 127 people died of storm-related causes in New Orleans–area hospitals (2008, 6). Many of these deaths were related to the prolonged power outage and lack of sanitation following the storm. It is likely that many of these deaths were related to prolonged exposure to heat, which can exacerbate underlying conditions. This same process likely caused the deaths of hundreds of people in Puerto Rico after Hurricane Maria in 2017.

Brian Stone explains how the body's thermoregulation system works and highlights what he calls the "central paradox" of heat-related deaths: "Many victims succumb to heat exhaustion or heat stroke during the night, when temperatures are lower than during the day" (2012, 4). He explains that under normal circumstances, a person is exposed to heat during the day and the body can recover at night. If there are above average temperatures during the night as well, "the body may not be afforded sufficient time to recover from heat exposure during a 24-hour period." The elderly, whose bodies are less able to regulate body temperature, are particularly sensitive to prolonged heat exposure.

> This is particularly true for vulnerable populations who lack access to air conditioning during the nighttime hours. If the body continues to perspire during the night as a person sleeps, the heart must continue to function at elevated levels and fluids must continue to be replenished. A failure to do so, particularly over a string of several days during a heat wave, can result in gradual increase in the body's core temperature. If this temperature increases beyond a very limited range—4 to 5 degrees—the likely result is death. (Stone 2012, 4)

Individuals who have an impairment of their cardiovascular system are particularly at risk of dehydration and death.

Sandy: Example of Helen Gatanis (Who Lived Alone and Would Not Evacuate)

This story demonstrates a common social pattern in the United States, namely, that many adult children live far away from their elderly parents and there are an increasing number of older individuals living alone without strong social networks (Gibson and Hayunga 2006). This story also shows again the multiple difficulties of evacuating someone with Alzheimer's disease (Christensen 2012; Christensen, Richey, and Castaneda 2013).

After Hurricane Sandy struck New Jersey and New York in October 2012, JoNel Aleccia, a staff writer for NBC, published an online article entitled "Confusion in the Storm: Alzheimer's Patient Refused to Evacuate" (2012). In this article, Aleccia described the dilemma faced by Senior Helpers as they attempted to safely provide care to Helen Gatanis, a woman in her eighties diagnosed with middle-stage Alzheimer's disease. Gatanis lived on her own in New Jersey. As is the case with many families, her son lived across the United States, in California.

Senior Helpers was hired on a part-time basis to assist Gatanis with her basic in-home needs four hours a day. When Hurricane Sandy threatened, Senior Helpers staff attempted to find Gatanis a temporary nursing home placement where she could safely weather the storm. They were able to transport Ms. Gatanis there; however, once in the nursing home, Gatanis became highly agitated, "distressed and combative." She was concerned about her cat, which remained in the home. Like Betsy and Joe Dunmore from chapter 1, Gatanis preferred her home, which was comfortable and familiar. A difference between Joe and Betsy's story and Gatanis's was that Gatanis did not have family or a legal guardian with her.

Aleccia notes that there are legal limitations to evacuating people; "there was no [legal] way to force Gatanis to stay" because despite her middle-stage Alzheimer's diagnosis, "she is competent to make such decisions" (2012). The article explains that "rather than upset her more, caregivers took her back home to wait out the storm." The caregivers indicated that Gatanis did not understand the risks that she was facing because when they handed her food and a flashlight, Gatanis inquired, "Why am I going to need my flashlight?" The caregivers did not stay with Gatanis for the duration of the storm.

This story, fortunately, has a happy ending because Helen Gatanis survived Hurricane Sandy without injury or illness, even though the Senior Helpers caregivers were unable to reach her for two days after the storm due to downed trees and power lines (though they may have asked local law enforcement to check on her).

Gatanis's situation, and the challenges faced by Joe and Betsy, point to an area of growing concern for emergency planners and informal caregivers: dementia of the Alzheimer's type is a progressive disease, which affects decision-making capacity and performance of functional activities of daily living over time. One of the hallmarks of the disease is the decline of executive function, which leads to poorer decision-making capacity and diminished judgment (Fink 2012). These abilities are crucial in planning response to risk (Schinka, Brown, and Proctor-Weber 2009). Alzheimer's disease and related disorders (ADRD) impact disaster planning because when executive functioning is impaired so is judgment when deciding how to respond to the risks associated with an upcoming hurricane (Stopford et al. 2012; Mayhorn 2005). In the middle and late stages, this disease can impair judgment to the point that an individual is unable to pick out weather-appropriate clothing. Sadly, many individuals who leave their home unaccompanied by a caregiver during extreme weather events die of exposure such as hypothermia or dehydration (Robinson et al. 2007).

It is unclear if Gatanis ultimately lost power during or after Hurricane Sandy, and if she did, how she kept warm in the cold days following the hurricane. I contacted the author, JoNel Aleccia, by email on February 22,

2014, to find out if she had more information on whether Gatanis had lost power. She did not have this information.

This is an important point to follow because another news article, by Sheri Fink of the *New York Times*, documented the sharp spike in hypothermia cases in emergency departments in the weeks following Hurricane Sandy (Fink 2012). This was especially true in early November 2012, when the nor'easter Nemo blew through the same area that Sandy had ravaged weeks before.

Post-Sandy Hypothermia

In total, there were 117 deaths as a result of Hurricane Sandy in New York, New Jersey, and Pennsylvania, and the mean age of those who died was sixty ("Deaths Associated with Hurricane Sandy" 2013). Fink reported that data were collected from patient records from those presenting to emergency departments following the blizzard that struck after Hurricane Sandy. The official count of hypothermia cases in New York was only sixty-five; however, it is thought to be an underrepresentation of the actual numbers because "the figure also did not reflect the much larger number of people whose underlying heart and lung problems had worsened in cold environments" (Fink 2012, para. 12).

This observation is important because it points to the environmental triggers of underlying disease, including interacting diseases that are identified as a syndemic. These individuals might have presented to the emergency room in respiratory distress or complaining of "chest pain" rather than "being cold" or "freezing," even if hypothermia was a triggering factor. Older individuals are especially vulnerable to extreme weather events because, as discussed earlier in this chapter, the body's ability to regulate internal temperature decreases as we age.

Fink pointed to another type of exposure that people might encounter as they try to keep warm: carbon monoxide poisoning from the use of gas stoves or gasoline-powered generators running inside the home. Again, because of metabolic changes, elders are more sensitive to toxins and environmental stressors. It has been well established that older individuals are sensitive to environmental exposures. In one study, Risher et al. explain that

> as a part of the aging process, the body gradually deteriorates, and physiologic and metabolic limitations arise. Changes that occur in organ anatomy and function present challenges for dealing with environmental stressors of all

kinds, ranging from temperature regulation to drug metabolism and excretion. (2010, 135)

Risher and his colleagues go on to argue that "the elderly are not just older adults, but rather are individuals with unique challenges and different medical needs than younger adults" (2010, 135). As the climate continues to be disrupted and more extreme weather events occur (i.e., stronger hurricanes and changes in overall weather patterns become more common), the physical and social conditions that conspire to make elders more vulnerable are likely to increase. These conditions need not be a death sentence, even during disasters (see chapter 7). We have the tools to mitigate many of the underlying vulnerabilities that lead to mortality.

ECOSYNDEMIC: TEMPERATURE VULNERABILITY

If vulnerability is considered normal and deaths as expected (see Fjord 2007) are overlooked, these intersecting factors can be identified as ecosyndemic. The **health conditions** involved in this ecosyndemic include the underlying chronic diseases, disabilities, or general frailty that can present in older populations, especially the oldest-old. These includes both bodily and mental health conditions. The **social conditions** include the increasing number of elders with impairments who are living alone, separate from family members, the large number of elderly on low fixed incomes, exclusionary practices (discussed below), and the relative lack of support for the elderly during and after disasters. The **ecological** and **ecosocial** factors at play in this ecosyndemic include anthropogenic extreme weather events and the nature of the built environment (e.g., lack of planning for flood surges and intense development in vulnerable coastal areas). Interaction among these three factors—a set of health conditions, a set of social practices and structures of inequality, and a set of environmental changes that reflect human activity—constitutes what might be called the Elderly Health Ecosyndemic.

SUMMARY

This chapter outlines the difference between normal aging and disease conditions and explains how those conditions can be exacerbated by climate change–related weather events. Alzheimer's disease is used to show how a condition associated with older age can affect a family's ability to respond to extreme weather events. Hurricanes in the United States are an example of such weather-related events, though many of these lessons can be applied to other events, including heat waves, prolonged freezing, and wildfires.

Chapter Seven

The Expected Dead: Bioethics, Vulnerability, and Expected Loss

While I huddled with my family at a hotel in Orlando, I learned that my neighbor "Liz" also evacuated with her two children before Hurricane Irma hit South Florida in September 2017. We communicated to check on each other. Her husband, "John," however, stayed home with his elderly father, "Dan." Dan used oxygen, which relies on an electronic pump. He had difficulty getting out of bed and needed assistance with most of his ADLs. He only moved in with the family four months before Hurricane Irma hit and it had not occurred to Liz or her husband then to sign him up for a special needs shelter. They were new to caregiving. By the time Hurricane Irma looked as if it was going to make a direct hit to their area and they started to make inquiries, it was too late to sign up for a special needs shelter. It would be incredibly difficult to relocate Dan anywhere because of his mobility problems.

After the storm, they agreed to let me formally interview them about their experiences. As the storm had hit on Sunday night, John described it as loud, and tree branches were snapping. Water flooded the streets, edging its way up the driveways. When the eye of the storm gave a temporary pause, John left his father's side and waded out into the street to check on the storm drains in the street. They were blocked with downed branches and leaves. He quickly dragged the branches away and watched the water drain, like water in a bathtub drain. John was back in his home with Dan by the time the other side of the storm arrived. As soon as the storm passed, John set up the generator. They are fortunate that they, like my family, could afford a generator and gas. Our community was exceedingly lucky: the storm hit at a slightly different angle than was predicted; the storm surge waters from the nearby river never hit our neighborhood. During Hurricane Katrina, many areas were not fortunate, and the flooding was largely unexpected.

THE EXPECTED DEAD

Mortality patterns and how they are reflected in the popular media can give insight into who is valued in a society. Some of the first academic research looking at the deaths resulting from Hurricane Katrina (2005) were published by Brunkard, Namulanda, and Ratard three years following the hurricane (2008). In 2009, another group of researchers, Jonkman et al., evaluated the same topic, though strictly within the state of Louisiana (the hurricane affected Alabama as well). As the popular media translated the scientific language of Jonkman's paper into a less formal format (for the lay public), cultural assumptions filtered into the reporting in a much more obvious way. Journalist Mark Schleifstein inserted his own interpretation of the researchers' findings, stating that they "jibe with common sense. The dead were overwhelmingly old," as if it were to be expected that the elderly bear the greatest burden of a disaster (Schleifstein 2009, para. 1).

Jonkman's team compared the deaths due to Hurricane Katrina to the 1953 flood in the Netherlands, which had "a higher vulnerability of elderly" because of "large-scale and more unexpected flooding" (2009, 686). The team explained that surviving such unexpected flooding "will be related to individual endurance, which is generally less for elderly" (2009, 686). They explained that over half of the recovered bodies were found in their homes. Schleifstein interpreted the findings by writing: "Neither race nor gender made anyone more likely to die, only a *failure to evacuate* and a location near a levee breach" (emphasis mine). While Schleifstein does acknowledge that evacuation was an "arduous" undertaking and not everyone was able to evacuate "quickly enough," he implicitly puts the blame for their death on the victims themselves (2009). For example, he writes that "the data reinforces the dire need for continuous improvement in the government's evacuation apparatus, particularly for the area's frailest, poor and *often hardest-to-motivate* residents" (emphasis mine). While acknowledging that the government needs to improve its response to assist the elderly and disabled, he also says the elderly and disabled lack motivation. Though research does suggest that older individuals are less likely to evacuate, they ought not be written off as lazy or simply lacking motivation (Eisenman et al. 2007; Christensen, Richey, and Castaneda 2013; Dash and Gladwin 2007). As demonstrated by my neighbors' experiences (above), there are real barriers for the frail and poor, such as access to accessible transportation, far beyond lack of motivation. If our neighborhood, which is upper middle class, had flooded with John and Dan trapped in their home, would Dan's death have been shrugged off as "common sense"?

VULNERABILITY AND EXPECTED LOSS

Though anthropologist Lakshmi Fjord accepts that the vulnerability concept in disasters was meant to highlight the social causes of differential burden during disasters, she argues that it may now serve as a justification of loss among vulnerable populations:

> The concept of vulnerability, as it is used in disaster rhetoric, may inadvertently reconstitute categories of persons for whom "expected losses" will occur. Intended to foreground the relationship between existing sociopolitical and economic inequalities and disproportionate losses after disasters, the vulnerability concept now fuels a hermeneutics of expectancy. (Fjord 2007, 60)

In Fjord's view, the vulnerability concept is at risk of being warped; rather than being used as a tool to examine the underlying, root causes of unequal access to safe housing, transportation, and healthcare, the vulnerability might instead be used to justify disproportionate losses among differing populations. Like the idea that elderly people are more likely to die during a disaster is just "common sense," she asserts that the concept of "vulnerability" can create a self-fulfilling prophecy of disproportionate loss among populations that are "expected" to suffer (2007).

Fjord uses critical disability theory to consider the response and documentation of disability during the aftermath of Hurricane Katrina. She analyzes the US House of Representatives Katrina Report on the media coverage "that led to the militarized responses in New Orleans" (2007, 49; "A Failure of Initiative" 2006). Within this document she considers the images produced from Katrina that created a skewed public perception of race, danger, and disability. She argues that these iconic images are presented without consideration of how exclusionary disaster planning practices contribute to the disproportionate deaths borne by black people, the frail elderly, and people with disabilities. These exclusionary practices, she posits, are the factor that creates the true disablement of these populations. However, public images do not present this critique. Instead, they normalize the suffering experienced by these marginalized populations. "They are the 'expected' dead, whose infirmities and age are imagined as the cause of their deaths. Through a critical disability lens, these images narrate instead the epistemology of a disaster bioethics based on 'one size fits all' disaster paradigms" (Fjord 2007, 49).

In other words, the public (much like Schleifstein) sees a person's age and need for a wheelchair as the causes of death. It is a fact that policy has not incorporated the needs of elderly populations into disaster planning priorities. A person is not disabled by a physical impairment alone. In such cases, it is the social environment that is more disabling than the impaired body of the individual. This is known as the social model of disability. The social model distinguishes between an impairment and a disability. An impairment or **disability** "is the functional limitation within the individual caused by physical, mental or sensory impairment" ("Constitution of Disabled People's International" 1993, Preamble). A **handicap** "is the loss or limitation of opportunities to take part in the normal life of the community on an equal level with others due to physical and social barriers" (1993, Preamble). The social model therefore emphasizes societal reactions to an impairment, with the term "handicap" calling attention to the oppression people with impairments experience because of prejudicial attitudes and discriminatory action (including a lack of access to buildings) (Oliver 1996). This is an important distinction because it reveals the importance of the social dimensions of disability, a corrective to our tendency to focus on the physical aspects of those labeled as disabled. Many individuals with a disability can function within society as long as there are alterations made to restrictive environments. Wheelchair users, for example, can function in the workplace if there are curb cuts and elevators that allow them access.

Some individuals require assistance with daily activities only once or twice a day. Policies that exclude the needs of vulnerable populations during disasters can be disabling, if not life threatening. Fjord implicitly references the social model of disability when she argues that disaster planning policies are disabling large segments of the population because they are seen as not "normal" and as "special needs" (Fjord 2007). While researchers need to be aware that some laypersons (e.g., politicians, journalists) might use the concept of vulnerability as a shortcut for explaining disproportionate loss, it is still an essential concept. It is the role of the research to critically examine root causes and structural violence and help the lay populations to connect the dots between these concepts and disproportionate loss during disasters.

Fjord and Manderson build on the critique of disasters and vulnerability in "Anthropological Perspectives on Disasters and Disability: An Introduction" (2009). They reference the "social model of disability" by locating the source of disablement in social practices and policy, outside of physical impairment. Rather, they argue that "vulnerable persons" ought to be conceptualized as being in "vulnerable situations." Citing Wisner et al.'s concept of "shifting vulnerabilities," they posit that vulnerability is a situation "which people move in and out of over time" (Wisner et al. 2004). The benefit of conceptualizing vulnerabilities as shifting, according to Fjord and Manderson, is that it allows theorists to "split apart the embodied or social characteristics of an individual or group from the social situation that cause differential burdens of harm because of barriers that deny them access to social and material resources" (2009, 67). The concept of shifting vulnerabilities is particularly helpful because a disease, such as Alzheimer's, also shifts over time, thereby changing a person's relationship to the social and policy environment. Fjord and Manderson also argue that the population at large can benefit from an expansion of disaster response services, not just "special needs populations" (2009, 64). FEMA is now requiring that all shelters, not just special needs shelters, be equipped to accommodate people with functional disabilities:

> Children and adults with disabilities have the same right to services in general population shelters as other residents. Emergency managers and shelter planners have the responsibility of planning to ensure that sheltering services and facilities are accessible. The decisions made in the planning process determine whether integration or segregation occurs during response. ("Guidance on Planning for Personal Assistance Services" 2010, 8)

Some state counties have balked at the cost and staff power that is necessary to make this transition, should it require a generator in each shelter and trained staff (Adams et al. 2011, 254). Furthermore, it may be difficult to find enough volunteer nurses to staff all the shelters in an area since many nurses are required to report to duty for their primary employer.

Nonetheless, the social model of disability is a powerful perspective that has shifted social policy to become more inclusive for individuals attempting to enter the work market and has increased accessibility standards. Certainly, from an ethical and social justice standpoint, all emergency shelters should be ADA compliant; however, elders, especially frail elders and those with age-related chronic illnesses or disabilities, should have options for specialized and appropriate support during disasters. For example, all Red Cross and county shelter volunteers should be trained in the unique needs of people with disabilities, including cognitive impairment; additionally, during disasters, special needs shelters that accept and are trained to work with people with Alzheimer's disease or a related dementia might provide a slightly less chaotic and more supportive environment than conventional shelters.

ASSISTANCE AFTER HURRICANES: FAILING OUR ELDERS

Continued challenges faced by elders who were evacuated before, during, or after Hurricane Katrina reflect cracks in the system. Anthropologists Adams, Kaufman, Van Hattum, and Moody present the plight of nearly 23,000 people who evacuated to the Astrodome in Texas after Hurricane Katrina.

> Here and elsewhere, medical personnel and shelter volunteers found that dozens of elderly were demented, had severe physical and mental impairments, and/or were gravely ill and needed immediate transfer to more medically sustainable surroundings. That was not always possible. (Adams et al. 2011, 254)

Without mechanisms in place to address the needs of individuals with physical and cognitive impairments, many of these individuals did not survive. The most vulnerable were those without (or separated from) family or social networks. "Others—without family, resources, or the wherewithal to obtain help—languished in shelters across the US, falling into poorer health and sometimes dying before their families could find them" (Adams et al. 2011, 254). The authors also point to policy deficits, which "lacked effective communication systems for locating displaced (or dead) persons" (2011, 255). When a person with an Alzheimer's disease diagnosis is surrounded by their social network, there is an increased chance that someone will help advocate for necessary care. Social networks can assist individuals to navigate the complicated process of recovery. For example, one participant reported that

> older people without family, who were incapable of managing the heavy demands of bureaucratic paperwork in order to receive insurance payments, Road Home monies, or Small Business Administration funds to rebuild, were overwhelmed, and many simply "gave up": they died because of depression

and they are not getting their money for the property, the right deal, or no deal. (Adams et al. 2011, 254)

The primary finding and concern of these researchers is that there is a "lack of government infrastructure for caring for evacuees, particularly the elderly" (Adams et al. 2011, 254). Wells echoes Adams et al.'s concern about the indirect deaths linked to Hurricane Katrina, especially among the elderly:

> Katrina is blamed directly for the deaths of 132 people in St. Bernard Parish . . . an elderly, infirm man found in the lap of his dead elderly wife who would not leave him behind; and 35 elderly residents of St. Rita's Nursing Home. But that hardly tells the tale. If you spend any time at all among residents, everyone has a story of deaths that, though not statistically tied to Katrina, they put into the Katrina column. These include many ill and infirm people who, separated from their doctors and medicine for far too long, died days or weeks or months afterward, never having fully recovered. It includes scores of the elderly who, seeing their homes destroyed beyond reclamation, simply gave up wanting to live. Ricky Robin himself had such a story. . . . After surveying the loss of his house, many of his prized boat carvings, and his way of life, [Ricky's father] took his own life in January 2006. He was seventy-five years old. (Wells 2008, 201)

The failure to include mechanisms for securing the safety of the most vulnerable populations, anthropologists (among others) argue, is rooted in a "one size fits all" or "greatest good" paradigm. Fjord argues that the "one size fits all" disaster paradigm prioritizes able-bodied individuals with the means to prepare and evacuate if needed. This excludes any person "who *temporarily or permanently* cannot see, hear, move, cognize, and cope during and after disasters, who has dependent kin, no cash or bank account, nowhere to go and no way to get there if they did" (Fjord 2007, 53, emphasis mine).

TRIAGE SYSTEMS: OFFICIAL AND UNOFFICIAL

Certainly, the "greatest good" paradigm (also known as utilitarianism, as coined by Jeremy Bentham and John Stewart Mill) requires that *someone* (or some group) decide *who counts as the majority worth saving* and who is designated as the *minority, worth sacrificing*. Like Fjord, Sheri Fink questions the concept of the "greatest good" when applied to disaster scenarios: "But what does the 'greatest good' mean when it comes to medicine? Is it the number of lives saved? Years of life saved? Best 'quality' years of life saved? Or something else?" (Fink 2013). Fink asked this question specifically about the triage systems used in hospitals after Hurricane Katrina and, later, Hurricane Sandy (Fink 2009a, 2012, 2013).

Both Lindy Boggs and Memorial (Baptist) hospitals had an unusually high number of deaths compared to other hospitals in New Orleans: nineteen patients died at Lindy Boggs and forty-five at Memorial. At Memorial, doctors were suspected of euthanizing patients after the storm, even as evacuation efforts were beginning to be resolved (Fink 2013). Fink suggests that part of the problem with the evacuation from these two hospitals (even though they had resources that other hospitals, such as the VA, did not) was with the implementation of the triage system. Triage is the process used by medical staff during emergencies to identify and categorize people who are the least injured or ill and those who are the most injured or ill. "Triaging victims requires selecting some to receive treatment before others" (Coleman et al. 2011, S112). This process is used to allocate essential medical services to those most in need. For example, when I worked in emergency rooms (ER) as a young woman (as an emergency medical technician), there was a nurse assigned to triage, screening people coming to the ER. If someone was having chest pain, a symptom of a potential heart attack, they were immediately admitted. If someone had stubbed their toe, they waited until the person with chest pain was treated, even if the person with a toe injury had arrived first. During **mass casualty incidents** (MCIs), however, the demand for services can exceed the supplies available. Examples of an MCI can range from a bus or train accident to an influenza pandemic. To avoid overwhelming the system, a "reverse triage" is implemented: rather than giving priority to those who are the most ill or injured, services are provided only to those most likely to survive (O'Laughlin and Hick 2008; Sprung et al. 2013). During Katrina, reverse triage was implemented at several hospitals, though without clear protocols on who was "unsavable," while resources remained and as evacuation efforts were under way (Fink 2013; Okie 2008).

Two sources recount the triage protocols that took place at Memorial and Lindy Boggs; both are the result of extensive interviews with staff. The first source is the result of a committee investigation that took place immediately after Hurricane Katrina ("A Failure of Initiative: Select Bipartisan Committee to Investigate the Preparation for and Response to Hurricane Katrina," 2006), and the second was the result of investigative journalism by Sheri

Fink (*Five Days at Memorial: Life and Death in a Storm-Ravaged Hospital*, 2013).

The following is Fink's description of how triage was implemented at Memorial Hospital:

> Doctors and nurses settled on a new method for categorizing the many more than one hundred remaining Memorial and LifeCare patients as they were brought downstairs. They were divided into three groups to help speed the evacuation. Those in fairly good health who could sit up or walk would be categorized "1's" and prioritized first for evacuation. Those who were sicker and would need more assistance were "2's." A final group of patients were assigned "3's" and were slated to be evacuated last. That group included those whom doctors judged to be very ill and also, as doctors had agreed on Tuesday, those with [do not resuscitate] orders. (Fink 2013, 135)

Lindy Boggs Hospital implemented a triage system for evacuation as well. In this case, the primary triage decisions were made by emergency medical responders outside the hospital, rather than the doctors within.

> With no helipad and no assurance of ambulances a boat ride away on dry ground, hospital staff at first ferried only able-bodied non-patients from Lindy Boggs. On Wednesday, firefighters arrived and began directing drivers of the small dinghies and pleasure boats to take patients to a berm by a nearby post office to be picked up by helicopters. The roughly 150 patients were divided into categories: A, B, and C. Some doctors and nurses thought the C's, the most critical patients, should be rescued first. But the doctors and firefighters in charge decided to leave them for last. The concern might have been that there would not be medical care for them at the drop points. . . . Reporter Hoda Kotb asked firefighter Chris Shamburger the reason for the triage protocol. He offered little explanation: "that's the way things are done." (Fink 2013, 371)

During MCI events, emergency responders are trained to respond using the reverse triage system. Whether these systems were the best way to prioritize people in a disaster situation remains controversial, as does the dosage of medication given to many of those who were not prioritized. Some of the people who were included in this category were not particularly ill before Hurricane Katrina but needed some maintenance care. As the heat increased during the power outages after the storm, conditions worsened. During and after Hurricane Katrina, those who needed the least assistance were explicitly considered most worth saving. Those with more medical needs, even if a person's disability or illness was only temporary, were considered less worthy of evacuation.

Reverse triage is an ethically fraught concept. Though it has an important role in maintaining the function of medical services during an MCI, those doing the assessment must be trained to make the best decisions possible. People must also be reassessed frequently to evaluate if conditions have changed over time. Research on the allocation of respirators in hospitals has shown that there is very little consistency in the reverse triage process (Christian et al. 2009; Fink 2009b, 2010). Other research has demonstrated that (often unconscious) racial bias filters into the provision of care (Avenanti, Sirigu, and Aglioti 2010; Xu et al. 2009; Hoffman et al. 2016).

WHO GETS FLOODED?

Triage can unofficially take place at the government level as more affluent (and often, less racially diverse) areas are prioritized for disaster response. Hurricane Katrina was not the first time that more marginalized areas of New Orleans were "sacrificed" to save the more affluent areas (Cordasco et al. 2007). During the 1927 Mississippi River flood, New Orleans was likely to be inundated. Rather than allow the affluent downtown area to flood, officials intentionally damaged the levees in such a way that they would only flood the poorer areas, predominantly populated by black farmers. A 1927 issue of *Science* magazine described the scene as follows:

> The dykes are strengthened, inhabitants are notified. But along the lower Mississippi many thousands of people are Negro farmers and laborers and their families, people who often stick to their homes. . . . Many of these river dwellers, even if they have escaped with their lives, have now seen their homes wrecked. They have lost their best chance to plant their cotton and other crops. ("The Mississippi Flood and Flood Predictions" 1927, 3)

What the *Science* article does not mention is that these floods were selective, caused by a "controlled break" of the New Orleans levees (Cordasco et al. 2007). This event was the result of white leaders in New Orleans deliberately targeting the most vulnerable in society who were dispensable: the black farmers and their families. This event has been preserved in the local memory. Researchers, such as Gregory Button (2006) and Cordasco et al. (2007) found that the long history of social, economic, and environmental injustice in this area was remembered after Hurricane Katrina: many hurricane survivors from the 9th Ward suspected the government had (again) intentionally flooded their area, as officials had done to their grandparents in the past. This institutionalized "utilitarianism," where people who are considered as less important are sacrificed to save those who are considered more important, remains largely intact in disaster response. It is important to emphasize that this is not strictly "utilitarianism" (greatest good for the greatest number). Instead, it is about whom the people in a position of power consider to be most valuable. In a capitalist society, that often translates into who produces the most for those in power, or who looks the most like those in power.

PUERTO RICO AFTER HURRICANE MARIA

Though Puerto Rico is a US territory, it received a far slower disaster response and much less news coverage than Hurricanes Harvey and Irma (Bump 2017). While there are legitimate barriers to providing services to the noncontiguous United States, there are also legitimate concerns that racial bias is also a factor for the underwhelming response. Polls taken after Hurricane Maria revealed that at least 50 percent of Americans do not know that Puerto Rico is an American territory (DiJulio, Muñana, and Brodie 2017; Olivera 2017). In a time of heightened anti-immigrant sentiments, this can shape expectations of who is deserving of aid (Garcia-Navarro 2017; Lopez 2017; Onís 2018). Historically protectionist legislation, such as the Jones Act, takes on a punitive effect as residents wait for disaster relief (Onís 2018). While this act is usually waived (and eventually was on September 28, 2017), its waiver was delayed and only came after political pressure was placed on the Trump administration, and it was allowed to expire within a month (Zanona 2017). Fueling the suspicion that the Trump administration was treating Puerto Rico differently than other states were tweets from the president claiming Puerto Ricans "want everything done for them," implying they were lazy (Lopez 2017). The American Civil Liberties Union (ACLU) raised concerns about the response, claiming it demonstrated the second-class citizenship Puerto Ricans are subjected to (Onís 2018).

Despite claims that the death toll from Hurricane Maria was low (64) and the response a success in comparison to Hurricane Katrina, research indicates the death toll is closer to 1,052 (Jorgensen 2017; Robles 2017). The death toll matters "because it can influence aid and government response" (Sutter 2017).

SUMMARY

The aging population in the United States is growing, as are the numbers of people with age-related illnesses who are more vulnerable to hurricanes and the conditions that follow. The concept of vulnerability, however, can be warped to act as an excuse for excess deaths rather than a way to identify and mitigate the underlying problem. Lakshmi Fjord introduces the concept of the "expected dead," where excess deaths among the elderly and disabled are shrugged off as the natural order of things. This excuse is deployed, even if the vulnerability, such as an upper respiratory illness, is usually temporary; if the illness strikes during an inopportune time, such as after a hurricane, the result can be deadly. Fjord and Manderson (2009) suggest that researchers and first responders reframe the concept of vulnerability to "vulnerable situations" rather than "vulnerable people" (a concept first deployed by Wisner et al. 2004a). The combination of dense, largely older populations in coastal urban centers during a time of global climate change presents a cluster of risks that classify as an ecosyndemic (Baer and Singer 2014). As the climate is disrupted, stronger storms and unusual weather conditions are increasingly striking vulnerable areas, such as coastal areas or densely populated urban centers. The impact of these storms is exacerbated by rising sea levels. Hurricanes (and post-hurricane conditions) can, in turn, amplify underlying age-related illnesses. As there are now larger populations of elderly individuals living in vulnerable areas, emergency managers need to be aware of how environmental changes can amplify the impact of disease, creating clusters of suffering.

Chapter Eight

Ecosocial Conditions, Built Environment, and Population Geography

When I first moved to Florida, I made sure to live within a mile of the university campus I would attend. I would save money by not having to maintain a car or buy a parking pass. I would also get much-needed exercise walking or riding my bike to campus. I could pat myself on the back for not contributing extra CO_2 into the atmosphere.

Something that I had not realized, however, was that the city of Tampa was not built for pedestrians or bike riders; in fact, it was almost hostile to them; it has ranked within the top ten most dangerous places in the United States for pedestrians and cyclists for over a decade (Kitali et al. 2017). After paying my deposit for an apartment, I watched, in shock, as a person in an electric wheelchair drove down the busy street, toward the curb. I watched cars swerve around the person, sometimes crossing a double yellow line as they approached a blind corner. Later, I saw mothers pushing strollers along the same road. Along the side of the road was either dust or mud, so the wheels of the stroller and wheelchair would not function, forcing everyone to share the road with cars. Students had to travel along this road to get to bus stops that were not connected by a sidewalk, only the muddy, dusty walk-way. It remains this way as I write in 2017. There are bus stops, but they are in the mud or dust in most locations.

The risk of death or injury was not spread evenly across the population: people of color and the elderly were far more likely to be killed or injured while walking (Buehler and Pucher 2017; Venciana-Suarez 2017; Dumbaugh and Zhang 2013). Owning a car became a necessity for me. But I was one of the lucky ones: I could afford a car. Those who cannot afford a car or cannot drive are at greater risk for injury or death. More than once, my university mourned the death of a student, killed traveling between home and campus. In 2010, there were nine cyclist fatalities within the span of four months. But most of the fatalities were not students. *Most fatalities were older individuals* (Dangerous By Design 2016, 21).

This chapter addresses some of the ways in which population settlement patterns, such as urban sprawl and poor urban planning in the United States, have contributed to dependency on fossil fuels and high levels of CO_2 in the atmosphere. Second, it explores the built environment, such as roads, buildings, drainage pipes, and other infrastructure in which humans live. These features are not only affected *by* climate (such as a dam being overwhelmed by flooding) but can also have an impact *upon* climate and weather (dams can disrupt regular water flow, such as in the Everglades). In addition, risks associated with more specific settlement patterns, such as living in rural areas, megacities, and coastal areas, are examined.

The impact of the built environment and how humans can change cold-weather patterns also are addressed. Building codes for these different modes of living vary widely. Urban sprawl (the suburban development of areas on the periphery of a city) and the "urban heat island effect" (the trapping of heat in urban centers, which makes them significantly warmer than more rural areas) are examples of an interactive relationship between the built environment (fueled development policies) and the natural environment (influenced by topographical features, longitude, latitude, and overall climate).

While the urban heat island effect can be observed in nearly any large city, urban sprawl has been a favored form of development in the United States. Urban sprawl, some argue, is a major reason the United States is a dominant contributor to CO_2 emissions because it means longer commutes and, in general, larger, more energy-hungry homes (Gonzalez 2010). The urban heat island effect can also be observed in highly developed suburban areas, though it is not as extreme as in the densely populated urban centers. Urban and suburban areas both replace vegetation with impermeable, dark asphalt and roofing materials, both of which trap heat (Stone 2012). These areas remain warmer even in average temperatures and can easily reach dangerous levels during extreme weather events, such as heat waves. During prolonged hot weather, infrastructure can become stressed and fail, becoming a serious public health threat (Stone 2012; Stott, Stone, and Allen 2004).

There are also properties that are unique to individual cities. Densely populated coastal cities are particularly vulnerable to climate change due to rising sea levels and the potential for stronger storms. Megacities (cities with over eight million people), such as New York and Los Angeles, are difficult to evacuate when faced with a major storm (Kramer, Khan, and Jahn 2011). The population size and density combined with limited roadways can challenge evacuation efforts. Population density was the reason that a mandatory evacuation order was not issued for Houston before Hurricane Harvey (Wang, Wootson, and O'Keefe 2017).

Some elders are drawn to cities because there are programs and facilities that are designed to provide services to older populations. The places that make the provision of services more convenient can become traps during mass power outages. At the same time, rural areas can be among the last to have services restored. The failure of critical infrastructure, such as medical facilities, can contribute to loss of life, especially for vulnerable elders. Consequently, long-term care facilities must be incorporated into essential disaster planning services.

BUILDING CODES

Building codes, locations, and other aspects of the built environment can alter vulnerability to natural hazards. In the introduction, I described how Betsy struggled to install hurricane panels on her home in 2004, before multiple hurricanes struck Florida. She managed this with the help of a neighbor, who, unlike Betsy, did not have hurricane shutters on her home. Betsy's neighbor did not have shutters because her home was built several years before Betsy and Joe's home. When the neighbor's home had been built, different building regulations had been in place in the county. In general, Florida building regulations underwent major changes after 1992, the year Hurricane Andrew struck south of Miami (Tsikoudakis 2012; Kusisto and Campo-Flores 2017). Most building codes are regulated at the county level and older homes are not held to the same standards as newly built homes. It would be cost prohibitive to require all homeowners to retrofit their homes to meet changing safety standards every year.

Building codes and urban planning have substantial impact on a city's vulnerability and potential resilience in times of disaster. Newer structures that are built to withstand wind and flooding are less likely to sustain damage. This is especially important when evaluating critical infrastructure such as hospitals and nursing homes. Though some lessons were learned from the aftermath of Hurricane Katrina, there were still many shortcomings in New York's preparation and response to Hurricane Sandy.

There are other factors that contribute to vulnerability and risk based on characteristics of the built environment, including the designation of flood zones and evacuation areas, the maintenance of mitigation regimes such as levees, dikes, and storm drainage, and the design of evacuation routes leading away from threatened areas.

In contrast with urban areas, rural environments can lack infrastructure and support in the wake of a disaster. The Lake Okeechobee area in central Florida is a prime example of a relatively isolated, impoverished, and resource-bare area that is highly vulnerable to flooding should a hurricane directly hit the area (Zhang, Xiao, and Leatherman 2006). This area is highly dependent on agriculture, the sugar industry, which attracts migrant workers. Migrant workers and the multigenerational families who live in the area, many of whom have modest incomes, lack reliable transportation, and can therefore easily become stranded before or during a storm.

URBAN SPRAWL AND DEPENDENCE ON CARS

Urban sprawl helps to explain the United States' reliance on the automobile, energy-intensive housing, and the fact that US citizens are responsible for more per capita CO_2 emissions than any other country: "The United States emitted 19.6 tons of carbon dioxide for every one of its residents in 2005, while France emitted 6.2 tons; United Kingdom 8.8; South Korea 9.3; Japan 9.5; Germany 9.9" (Gonzalez 2010, 18). All countries listed have populations over 45 million.

George Gonzalez points to the late 1800s as the beginning of moderate urban sprawl, brought about by the advent of the electrically powered trolley (2010, 46). Even with the trolley, development was relatively compact and near city centers compared with the wide dispersal of suburban communities today. When the gasoline-powered automobile became more affordable and therefore more accessible in the 1920s, land developers saw it as a reason to develop land even further out (and increase their property value). Gonzalez uses Los Angeles as a classic example of this process. As privately owned automobiles replaced the public trolley systems and the suburban areas expanded horizontally, Los Angeles sprawled exponentially. Indeed, legislative analyst Bradford Snell accused car companies of deliberately destroying the trolley system to improve their sales (1974). It is now known as the smog capital of the United States (Gonzalez 2010, 13). In addition, it is a coastal megacity, potentially vulnerable to sea level rise and storms.

After the crash of the stock market in 1929, the federal government began to back policies that encouraged urban sprawl even further "through a program that guaranteed home loans for newly constructed housing on the urban periphery" (Stern 2010). These policies encouraged home construction on the outskirts of urban areas and without alternative transportation options, they also implicitly required that homeowners become car owners. In the 1950s, the federal government financed the highway system, further supporting the dominance of the automobile as the primary means of transportation.

In addition, as Gonzalez points out, homes in the suburbs tend to be larger than those in the city centers (e.g., apartments), requiring more energy to heat and cool them. These larger homes also create a demand for more appliances (such as refrigerators and air conditioners) and furniture, which spurred the economy but also contributed to the high CO_2 emissions produced by the United States. Gonzalez directly connects the United States' continued support of urban sprawl development with its contribution to climate change:

> While urban sprawl in the United States serves to prop up the world economy, urban sprawl has a number of environmental costs associated with it. Firstly, horizontal urban expansion destroys open space and wilderness. . . . Urban sprawl also draws down finite fossil fuels at a prodigious rate. . . . This huge use of fossil fuels substantially contributes to the climate change phenomenon. These fuels are being consumed at such high rates that the carbon dioxide emitted by their burning cannot be benignly absorbed by the biosphere of the planet. (Gonzalez 2010, 18)

Europe, however, developed in a vastly different, more compact, manner than the United States. Gonzalez compares Belgium and the state of New Jersey, which though they "have similar land to population ratio and per capita income, per capita automobile ownership and use is substantially higher in New Jersey" (2010, 13). Gonzalez cites economic factors as the source of these differences: after World War II, Europe lacked resources for new housing stock and the Western European economies were not geared toward durable domestic goods (e.g., household appliances) as they were in the United States.

In Europe, trolleys were used to make urban transportation more efficient within and between cities, not to reach further outlying areas as was the case in the United States. Consequently, there are comprehensive rail systems in Europe today, while this is not the case in the United States. In addition, Europe does not have the capacity to produce the same extensive amounts of oil, coal, or natural gas; should European countries have adopted strategies like the United States, they would have been largely dependent on outside sources for heating and cooling homes in addition to transportation.

Gonzalez also points out that "in post–World War II era, the countries of Europe did not have the military and political capacity to intervene in the Middle East to ensure that the oil from this region amply flowed" (2010, 13). That the United States was no longer producing enough oil to sustain its domestic needs meant that it needed to use military intervention in oil-rich regions. The staggering cost of US military action in the Middle East since 1976 is estimated to be $7.6 trillion (and this does not account for the number of lives lost in the multiple "interventions" in which the United States has been engaged). Scholars, such as Hans Baer, draw attention to the "critical need for public transit in the era of climate change" (2016).

CITIES AS HEAT ISLANDS AND IMPACT ON HEALTH

As addressed above, the "urban heat island" effect can put city dwellers at greater risk for heat-related illnesses. Stone argues that, in the past, forest land cover (which reduces overall temperatures) was replaced by crops. Now, however, forests and other land cover are "displaced by the most hydrologically inert materials imaginable: concrete, asphalt, and roofing shingle" (2012, 100). Asphalt and concrete do not allow moisture to permeate the soil; as a result, natural cooling convection does not take place. The urban heat island can contribute to the failure of infrastructure during heat waves:

> Much like the human body, urban infrastructure can become stressed during prolonged periods of intense heat. It is the failure of infrastructure in the form of transportation and electrical power systems that can pose one of the most significant—and the least anticipated—threats of rising temperatures to urban environments. (Stone 2012, 5)

When infrastructure, such as electrical systems, fails, so does the ability to cool homes and public places.

Usually, heat events are predictable, which makes a certain level of planning possible. However, as has been observed numerous times, even in developed countries (such as Chicago in the United States in 1995 and in Europe in 2003), many, especially vulnerable elderly, still die in disproportionate numbers (Della-Marta et al. 2007; Poumadère et al. 2005). During the 2003 heat wave in Europe, eighty thousand excess deaths were recorded, compared to the 1998–2002 period (Robine et al. 2007). This heat wave affected women and people over the age of ninety-five disproportionately, 21 percent above the expected number for females, and 46 percent for the over ninety-five (Robine et al. 2007).

COLD WEATHER

As discussed in chapter 3, global warming can also bring colder temperatures to lower latitudes that are not as well equipped for such extremes (as seen in Alabama and Georgia during the winter of 2013–2014). In addition, as overall warmer temperatures cause greater water evaporation from the Gulf of Mexico and Atlantic Ocean, the amount of atmospheric moisture available to fuel winter storms, such as nor'easters, has been increasing.

Land use, such as extensive irrigation, can also affect winter temperatures. Stone gives the example of Florida's hard freeze in 1997, which devastated the orange groves (2012, 48–51). After multiple hard freezes, orange groves were relocated farther south in Florida. To accommodate the relocation, wetlands were drained. "Natural wetlands moderated falling temperatures by releasing heat energy absorbed during the day throughout the night, when temperatures reach their minimum" (Stone 2012, 48). When the wetlands were drained to make room for the relocated orange groves, the likelihood of hard freezes in the state increased. Crops can benefit from being downwind from a lake, known as the "lake effect" (2012, 50). The benefit is lost when wetlands are drained. Another lesson from this example is that though there might appear to be some initial benefits of a warming climate for agriculture (warmer temperatures leading to fewer hard freezes), it is ultimately detrimental; warmer temperatures overall can eventually stunt the growth of crops as lakes evaporate and temperatures swing to extremes (Solomon et al. 2007).

Though deaths were not reported during the 1997 freeze in Florida, cold weather events are responsible for the greatest number of weather-related deaths in the United States (followed by hot weather) (Kapur and Smith

2011). Cities with generally cooler weather tend to have the most deaths from both hot and cold weather extremes (2011). There are several factors that can render individuals more vulnerable to weather-related death, including (1) older age (over sixty-five), (2) living alone, (3) lower socioeconomic status, (4) lack of access to air-conditioning or heat, (5) taking multiple medications, and (6) multiple comorbid medical conditions (e.g., heart disease and diabetes).

MEGACITIES

There has been a global demographic shift; more people are living in cities than in rural areas. According to World Wildlife Federation International, "cities cover only 1% of the planet's surface," but they "use 75% of the world's energy and emit 75% of global greenhouse gases" (Kramer, Khan, and Jahn 2011, 6). Other researchers have noted that "as in industrialized countries more and more of the population becomes urbanized and the percentage of people with higher age increases continuously, the threat of temperature-related mortality will probably become more severe over the next decades" (Schneider et al. 2011, 128).

The IPCC identifies eight aspects of cities that can increase disaster risk and vulnerability and are relevant in the context of climate change:

1. The synergic nature of the city and the interdependency of its parts.
2. The lack of redundancy in its transport, energy, and drainage systems.
3. Territorial concentration of key functions and density of building and population.
4. Mislocation.
5. Social-spatial segregation.
6. Environmental degradation.
7. Lack of institutional coordination.
8. The contrast between the city as a unified functioning system and its administrative boundaries that many times impede coordination of actions. (Cardona and Van Aast 2012, 78)

Nearly twenty years ago, Juha Uitto, a social and economic geographer, wrote about the increased risk of megacities' exposure to natural hazards (1998). It is Uitto's assumption that the number of natural hazards will remain the same; however, exposure (structures, buildings, humans, and other entities at risk) and vulnerability (propensity to suffer loss) may have increased because of rapid urbanization, especially in coastal areas (1998). While the settlement patterns do increase exposure, climate change is increasing the frequency and intensity of many weather-related disasters (Klein, Nicholls, and Thomall 2003; Kunreuther, Michel-Kerjan, and Ranger 2012; Mallick, Ahmed, and Vogt 2017; Romieu et al. 2010).

As can be seen with the urban heat island effect, cities can both *affect* and *be affected by* climate change. Larger cities that contain eight million inhabitants or more are considered megacities, and institutional coordination within them can be complex (Allen et al. 2012).

In the United States, there are two megacities, both of which are located along the coasts: New York and Los Angeles. Hazards that threaten coastal megacities include (1) erosion of beaches and coastlines; (2) storm and wind damage; (3) flooding; and (4) salinization of surface waters (Klein, Nicholls, and Thomall 2003). A significant amount of America's older population is living in densely populated coastal areas, which makes them especially vulnerable to these threats.

COASTAL LIVING

In 2010, 39 percent (over 123 million people) of the US population lived in coastal shoreline areas (not including Alaska) ("The U.S. Population Living at the Coast" 2012). The coastal population has increased by 34.8 million people (39 percent increase) between 1970 and 2010 and is projected to continue to grow. NOAA warns that "this situation presents coastal managers with the challenge of both protecting coastal ecosystems from a growing population and protecting a growing population from coastal hazards" ("The U.S. Population Living at the Coast" 2012).

By 2050, people over the age of sixty-five will make up approximately 20 percent of the US population. Many of these people are likely to live in coastal areas. Florida is projected to have over 4.4 million people over the age of sixty-five by 2020 ("Florida Population by Age Group" 2016). In addition to large older populations, Florida has long stretches of coastal property and densely populated urban centers.

Living along the coast increases the likelihood of hurricane impact. Crowded cities built in coastal areas are not only popular retirement destinations (as was demonstrated by Betsy and Joe's story in chapter 1), but they are prone to greater damage to infrastructure during a disaster.

RURAL AREAS

While megacities are complex and therefore a challenge for coordinating mitigation and disaster response efforts, they do tend to have more resources and are given more priority in government spending than rural areas (Allen et al. 2012). The Lake Okeechobee area in Florida is an example of a rural area that is highly vulnerable to climate change–related disasters, especially hurricanes. Though not located directly on the Atlantic or Gulf of Mexico coast, the size and relatively shallow depth of Lake Okeechobee makes it particularly prone to storm surges (as took place in the 1928 hurricane). The inhabitants of the area tend to come from lower socioeconomic backgrounds and communities, even those located in the relatively wealthy Palm Beach County, and tend to be resource poor (Zhang, Xiao, and Leatherman 2006). Another potential concern are people living in rural areas who are without access to transportation. According to the 2000 census, there were 10.8 million households without cars in the United States ("Census Transportation Planning Products" 2011). This might not be a significant barrier to disaster response in cities that have public transportation options (though it continued to be a barrier in New Orleans). However, 1.1 million of these households without cars were in rural areas, which can make evacuation difficult before a disaster (2011). Moreover, having a driver's license sharply drops off after the age of seventy-five (Gibson and Hayunga 2006; Polzin, Pisarski, and Weinberger 2013). Older individuals, especially those over the age of seventy-five, who live in rural areas are at risk for prolonged isolation after disasters.

BUILDING CODES AND FLOOD ZONES

Local communities are the first line of defense in disaster preparation, response, recovery, and mitigation. Building codes are part of the mitigation process in the disaster cycle. Building codes are largely designated at a local level because different areas have different risks, but also different political landscapes. In areas that have extreme winters, building codes usually require roofs to be able to bear a heavy load of snow to prevent collapse. This kind of code is unlikely to be in place in Florida counties because it rarely snows. Florida, however, has a need for buildings that can withstand strong winds during a hurricane, and the building codes reflect that.

When Hurricane Sandy struck, nearly two-thirds of the damaged homes were located outside the predicted flood zones. This led to a vast redrawing of New York City's flood zone (Colvin 2012; Buckley 2013). The new flood zones added nearly 600,000 residents to evacuation zones (Gibbs and Holloway 2013). Evacuation of large cities such as New York is extremely difficult, and the local authorities advise against evacuating by car if there are other options available.

PLANNING FOR EVACUATION

In November 2012, Atkins Global, an engineering and planning consulting firm, presented a list of ten areas that it considered to be the most difficult to evacuate before a hurricane strike. These areas include (1) Southwest Florida (Naples area); (2) Tampa Bay, Florida; (3) Delaware, Maryland, Virginia peninsula; (4) New York City / New Jersey area; (5) Southeast Florida (Miami, West Palm Beach, the Keys); (6) Hampton Roads, Virginia; (7) New Orleans, Louisiana; (8) Galveston / Houston, Texas, areas; (9) Jacksonville, Florida; (10) Myrtle Beach, South Carolina.

The factors that contribute to the difficulty of evacuating Southwest Florida include the limited roadway escape capacity and high traffic areas. Before a storm, the traffic from southwestern Florida would likely be compounded by traffic from southeastern Florida and the Tampa Bay area. Furthermore, there is a large elderly population, a large mobile home community, and limited emergency sheltering. In addition, there are very few public transportation options that could take residents into safer areas. The limited evacuation routes (via freeways and lack of public transportation) are a common barrier for seeking safety in nearly all the areas named in the Atkins report.

DESIGNATING SHELTERS AND SAFE SPACES IN FLORIDA

In 2017, there were multiple problems with the emergency shelters during Hurricane Irma. There were reports that the schools lost power, ran out of food, and had no running water, creating unsanitary and potentially unsafe conditions (Bland 2017a, 2017b; Washington et al. 2017). David Hodges, an investigative reporter at NBC2 News, found that during Hurricane Irma at least five thousand people were sheltered in locations that had a 10 percent chance of flooding up to three feet (Hodges 2017b). This risk was known before the storm and the American Red Cross declined to run these shelters due to flooding concerns. Lee County Emergency Management opened the shelters anyway as the demand for shelters was great.

RECOVERY

The recovery efforts in Texas, Florida, and Puerto Rico in 2018 followed very different trajectories, largely because of geography and the building codes that guided development (Garcia-Navarro 2017). In Florida, Hurricane Andrew spurred a revamp of the building codes (Jacobo 2017). In the first chapter, I described how Betsy's home had hurricane shutters but her neighbor's did not. This was because her home was built after 1992 when Hurricane Andrew hit, but her neighbor's home was grandfathered in because it was built earlier. The updated building codes, like most areas, did not require older buildings to be updated. The building codes in Puerto Rico did not have such a revamp (Dooley 2017). Critical infrastructure, such as the electrical grid, was decimated after Hurricane Maria, cutting power to hospitals and nursing homes alike (Carabello and Shechet 2017; Francis 2017; Robles 2017). This is likely a major contributing factor to the surge in deaths identified after Hurricane Maria (Jorgensen 2017).

SUMMARY

Ecosyndemics include ecological and ecosocial factors, as well as social and health conditions. The built environment is part of the ecosocial, the intersection between ecology, the environment, and how people respond and build in those environments. Especially in large coastal cities, the built environment can amplify vulnerability to hurricanes. This is a growing problem, especially because large numbers of older individuals are living in urban areas. Long-term care facilities must be incorporated into essential disaster planning services. Rural environments can lack infrastructure while urban environments can intensify heat and be more difficult to evacuate. The failure of critical infrastructure, such as medical facilities, can contribute to loss of life, especially for vulnerable elders.

Chapter Nine

Social Conditions, Long-Term Care, and Disasters

DEATHS IN A FLORIDA NURSING HOME

Three days after Hurricane Irma, we do not have power. It is hot. In the nineties where we are (certainly could be worse). Sweat flows freely from our brows, but we are healthy, with no underlying cardiovascular disorders. We are middle aged; our bodies' thermoregulation systems work well. Our children's too. We can jump in the pool if it gets too hot. We have a generator that can keep us cooler at night. Those are all things that many frail elders cannot easily do, whether cared for at home or in a facility (Van Someren 2007). Maybe they do not have a generator. Generators are expensive and require maintenance, and many retired people are on a fixed income. In a skilled nursing facility, people depend on others to control the temperature.

My cell phone signal is weak. I can receive text messages, which use less bandwidth, but I cannot download news articles. I get news alerts though, so I see headlines. On Wednesday, September 13, I see the headline: "At Least 8 Dead after Irma Leaves Florida Nursing Home with No A/C" (Nedelman, Almasy, and Grinberg 2017). My heart sinks. I suspect it was preventable, but I cannot read the details. I know how vulnerable elders are to heat, especially if they have an underlying chronic illness. I know that under Florida statutes, skilled nursing facilities are required to have a generator as backup power to prevent deaths caused by excessive heat (Brown, Hyer, and Polivka-West 2007). Questions run through my head: Was their generator in a flood-prone area? Was the generator not hooked up to the air-conditioning

(AC)? Did they prioritize refrigerating the food instead of AC? I think back to the focus groups I helped to conduct in 2009, with over thirty nursing home administrators and nurses (working with Dr. Kathryn Hyer and Dr. Lisa M. Brown) (Christensen, Brown, and Hyer 2012). I thought of all the tough decisions Florida nursing home administrators told us about: what they weighed when deciding to evacuate or to shelter in place as a storm approached; how much fuel to keep on hand; where to store the generator (and how expensive it was to relocate one from a flood-prone area to a safer place); and how to train the staff for hurricane preparedness and aftermath.

My colleagues have done so much to learn about, support, and train skilled nursing and assisted living facility staff in Florida that it seems odd to me that administrators would not have anticipated this risk (Hyer et al. 2009; Christensen, Brown, and Hyer 2012). They send me more details, copying and pasting newspaper articles into an email so I can read the articles: that the Hollywood skilled nursing facility was near a hospital, that facility staff had been in contact with the Emergency Operations Center a few days earlier, said they were OK. By the next day, eight residents at the Rehabilitation Center at Hollywood Hills had died and a criminal investigation was being conducted (McMahon, Bryan, and Pesantes 2017). This was a primary example of how the ecosocial, health conditions, and social conditions interacted to amplify mortality, resulting in an ecosyndemic.

The next day, trucks from Kansas City, Kansas, restored power to our street and I was able to access more information. The death toll had risen to eleven people in the Hollywood nursing home (Sarkissian 2017). One of the residents had an internal body temperature of 106 degrees at time of death (Shapiro and Jacobo 2017). Headlines began to emerge that though the governor of Florida, Rick Scott, had distributed his cell phone number to nursing home administrators, when staff at the Rehabilitation Center at Hollywood Hills called that number, they say they were ignored (Fowler, Jacobo, and Shapiro 2017). Later, it was reported those voicemails were erased (Ostroff 2017; Swenson 2017). The governor responded to the deaths by instituting a new rule for inspections of generators at nursing facilities (Richmond 2017).

Within three weeks of Hurricane Irma, most of Florida had power restored. After four months, the island of Puerto Rico has not been as fortunate; as of this writing, some reports say that some areas will not have power restored within a year (Francis 2017; Carabello and Shechet 2017; Feere-Sadurni, Robles, and Alvarez 2017; Nedelman 2017; Chaney 2017). When so many hospitals and nursing homes remain without power, it is difficult to imagine the situation of elders who live in the community (Brown, Hyer, and Polivka-West 2007).

SKILLED NURSING FACILITIES

Though most elders live in the community, hospitals and skilled nursing facilities do house large numbers of vulnerable people and they are expected to keep these populations safe (Hyer et al. 2009). It is shocking when these safe havens fail in their task during disasters. As the data from Hurricane Katrina suggest, even with professionally trained staff, elders can still suffer the greatest deleterious effects of a hurricane. The reasons for this are multi-faceted (and will be explained in more detail in the following chapter). Regulations for long-term care, such as assisted living and skilled nursing facilities, vary from state to state, though the underlying vulnerability of elders remains similar (Brown, Hyer, and Polivka-West 2007; Hyer et al. 2009; Achenbach, Hauslohner, and Sullivan 2017; "Caring for Vulnerable Elders During a Disaster" 2007).

Rather than providing acute care (such as an emergency room), nursing homes are designed to provide long-term care. Long-term care requires medical services that sustain life, including assistance with medications and minor medical procedures, such as dressing changes, and assistance with hygiene. Nursing home residents often require electrical-powered equipment, such as respirators, compressed oxygen, IV pacers, and pacers for feeding tubes, to keep them healthy and comfortable. Brown and her colleagues found that although nursing homes provide essential services, there is a wide variation in codes and regulations concerning emergency backup power for skilled nursing facilities. Loss of power is one of the primary reasons that facilities are forced to evacuate *after* hurricanes (2007).

The federal Centers for Medicare and Medicaid Services (CMS) oversees federal standards for nursing homes in the United States, including emergency preparedness and response. Unlike hospitals and fire departments, nursing homes are *not* always automatically considered to be essential facilities, and therefore are not always prioritized for power restoration after a hazard (Brown, Hyer, and Polivka-West 2007). Though the importance of designating skilled nursing facilities as a priority for power restoration was highlighted at the National Nursing Home Hurricane Summit in 2007, a decade later, residents were still dying from complications of loss of electricity

(Shapiro and Jacobo 2017). In 2017, another summit was called to address new rules requiring generators to be inspected in skilled nursing facilities (Klas 2017). It is unclear whether the new rule will address the fact that when nursing homes lose power, they are not usually required to have the air-conditioning connected to the generator (Brown et al. 2012, 2015).

Another summit is not likely to solve underlying issues because the risks facing nursing home residents and staff have been well established, as have several potential solutions. Here is what was known before the 2017 hurricane season: nursing homes are not automatically considered as a priority for power restoration after a storm, which can be a reason for forced evacuation after a hurricane strikes. Lack of power severely impacts a facility's ability to provide sanitary and safe medical support to their residents (Brown et al. 2012; Hyer, Polivka-West, and Brown 2008; Frank 2005). Additionally, the residents they serve are often older and more vulnerable to heat and cold, which may follow a hurricane event. In most states, nursing home administrators are tasked with developing relationships with the local emergency operations centers (EOCs) and ensuring that the local power companies know (1) that they are there; (2) they are providing essential medical services; and (3) they need to be on a priority power restoration list after disasters to keep the vulnerable elderly they serve safe. It is essential that nursing homes have strong disaster plans and build relationships with their local EOCs and the power companies that serve their areas before a storm hits (Wang, Wootson, and O'Keefe 2017). Emergency operations centers are a place where experts gather before, during, and after an emergency to monitor and disseminate information. They also coordinate responses and resources. Most emergency shelters and fire departments are connected to the county EOC during disasters through ham radios.

EVACUATING A SKILLED NURSING FACILITY

Evacuation can be costly for the facility, potentially unsafe, and at times, deadly for residents (McGraw and Ghebremedhin 2017). Before Hurricane Rita, a bus filled with elderly residents evacuating the storm caught fire (Hyer, Polivka-West, and Brown 2008; Thomas et al. 2010; Brown et al. 2012). This event was referenced in the decision not to issue a mandatory evacuation for the city of Houston, Texas, before Hurricane Harvey struck (Brown 2008; Hyer et al. 2009). At least one skilled nursing facility, La Vita Bella Nursing Home, flooded while twenty to twenty-five residents remained inside (Blanchard and Dosa 2009). Photographs circulated on social media showing residents sitting in wheelchairs with water up to their chests. Nursing home administrators must face a difficult choice when weighing risks: to shelter in place or evacuate before a storm.

Recent research demonstrates that evacuating can be stressful for residents with functional impairments; an increase in the number of deaths is documented months after a facility is forced to relocate in the wake of a storm (Dosa et al. 2007). When it is a safe and viable option, it is best for skilled nursing facilities to shelter in place. However, older facilities might not be able to withstand the high winds, and facilities located in flood zones need to evacuate or the consequences can be deadly. Strong disaster and mitigation plans can reduce the toll on both staff and residents (Cobb 2013; Wells 2008; Dosa et al. 2007). If a facility does not have proper storm shutters or safely located generators to run ventilators, laundry services, and air-conditioning (in at least some of the common areas), then evacuation should still be considered. Even in the best of circumstances, storms and their aftermath can pose significant challenges to nurses attempting to provide care to residents ("A Failure of Initiative" 2006).

Sheltering in place proved deadly during Katrina as was seen at St. Rita's Nursing Home and Lafon Nursing Home of the Holy Family (Cobb 2013). These facilities were located on relatively "high ground" that had not previously flooded during hurricanes (e.g., Hurricane Betsy, which made landfall in 1965, even before the levee system was in place) (Christensen, Brown, and Hyer 2012; Hyer et al. 2009). Because official mandatory evacuation orders were not issued for Jefferson County, where the nursing homes were located, the administrators made decisions based on previous experiences. During Hurricane Katrina, however, with the failure of the levee system these two occupied facilities were inundated and the choice to shelter in place resulted in many resident deaths (Kaye, Harrington, and Laplante 2010). The locus of blame, at least according the lawyer for St. Rita's, was the poor maintenance of the levee system rather than the decision making of the nursing home administrators (2010).

Disaster plans often change during or immediately after a storm due to unforeseen circumstances (such as damage to a building), and at times, nursing homes are forced to evacuate to nonclinical buildings like school gymnasiums or churches (Hyer et al. 2009; Brown, Hyer, and Polivka-West 2007). If evacuation is likely to become necessary, especially because of potential flooding, it is better to evacuate *before* a storm rather than during or after when resources are likely to be even scarcer and staff and residents are exhausted.

ASSISTED LIVING FACILITIES

Assisted living facilities (often referred to as ALFs), are homes, usually organized like apartments, where residents can receive moderate assistance with activities of daily living, such as giving medications or monitoring someone with mobility problems during a shower (to make sure there is not a fall). There are sometimes options for shared dining or having meals sent to the apartment.

Unlike most skilled nursing facilities, most ALFs are not eligible for Medicare or Medicaid coverage, and therefore must be paid for by private funds (Hyer et al. 2009). ALFs are not required to conform to the same sets of federal standards as skilled nursing facilities (Brown, Hyer, and Polivka-West 2007; Brown et al. 2015). As a result, their structure and the services provided can vary widely. While skilled nursing facilities are required to have a comprehensive disaster plan to provide continuous care for residents during a hurricane or other disasters, no such requirement exists for ALFs. This means that while some ALFs will provide sheltering assistance during hurricanes, others might require the residents to go stay with their family members during a storm. There have been reports, however, of residents refusing to evacuate before a storm, insisting on sheltering in the facility even if there was no available support staff (Pasch, Brown, and Blake 2011). Some residents may not have family members available to stay with during a storm. It is critical that ALFs have clear policies, contracts, and ongoing communication with families about how they plan to respond during weather-related disasters. They must also have contingency plans for residents who are unable or unwilling to evacuate the premises.

SHELL POINT AS AN EXAMPLE OF PROACTIVE PLANNING

Shell Point is a retirement community on the southwest coast of Florida that consists of transitional living options: independent living, assisted living, and skilled nursing. When one is no longer able to live completely independently and needs support, the resident can transition to a higher level of care "all covered by the same monthly maintenance fee" ("Shell Point Pricing" 2017).

This residence is located directly on the coast, extremely vulnerable to storm surges. A retired administrator at Shell Point, David Haverstick, said that, in 1995, when the need for expanded parking was pressing, one of the leaders suggested they also find a way to incorporate a storm shelter. They created a plan for a parking garage with a top level that could be converted to an emergency shelter during a cyclonic storm. It was designed so that shutters would come down to enclose the area and large fans could keep air circulating. Some perceived this additional design as an unnecessary expense, especially considering it could be years before a hurricane would force the shelter into use.

Every year during the first week of June, Shell Point featured a hurricane preparedness week. They would bring in a meteorologist to speak to the residents. They went over disaster kits, encouraging people to include medications and snacks.

In 2004, Hurricane Charley was predicted to hit the area. Before the storm, residents chose a reclining chair and packed one bag of belongings (about the size of a garbage bag). The chairs were moved to the shelter and set up a few days before the storm. The staff had sectioned out the area to reflect the different buildings where residents lived. They had arranged for a company to bring several portable toilets, which arrived before the storm.

About eight hours before the storm, residents were moved by buses, ambulance, or wheelchair into the building. They had food and water stocked. They had big fans that were run by generator, but not air-conditioning. "It was not comfortable," Mr. Haverstick told me. But it was safe. They had structured activities for the residents run by the staff. The residents slept in their chairs or on cots.

There were people on hospice in the shelter who died during the storm (but their deaths were expected). Though these residents were nearing the end of their life, it was judged unethical to abandon them. They were brought to the shelter so palliative care could continue. When they passed, their bodies were placed in body bags for the duration of the storm.

Some pets were allowed in the shelter but there were a lot of restrictions. Families of staff could come if they were able-bodied and could help assist with supportive care. About one-third of the staff did not come in, though they signed an agreement saying they would work in the event of a storm. They were worried about their own families. Those who came in displayed high morale. After the storm, the portable toilets were nearly full, and it was hot. The fans helped circulate air, but it was not the same as air-conditioning.

There were 125 units damaged during the storm, which could have resulted in fatalities. Except for some of those receiving hospice care, the residents fared well. There were no excess deaths. This planning, while initially unpopular due to cost, likely saved lives. However, access to such a community is prohibitive for many who are not independently wealthy. Most communities will depend on either county-run (like Bernice and her mother, Jean, see below) or Red Cross–operated shelters during storms.

In creating an on-site shelter above the storm surge and resistant to wind, Shell Point administrators avoided the greatest point of conflict most administrators face before a storm: whether to evacuate or to shelter in place (Hyer et al. 2009). They created a haven on-site for residents of all levels.

Since the 2004 storms, we as researchers working with long-term care facilities have learned much about how facilities can best support staff and encourage them to come in to work during a hurricane: allowing staff to bring families and pets, assigning a staff member to care for children, and providing rest areas for staff can reduce the conflict between dedication to work and dedication to families (Hyer et al. 2009; Dosa et al. 2007; Blanchard and Dosa 2009).

HOSPITALS

Hospitals are rarely ordered to evacuate, as they serve essential community services and are often structurally stronger than many nursing homes. As such, many people who require dialysis or other ongoing services come to the hospital in advance of the storm. There can be conflict, however; some skilled nursing facilities in Florida said hospitals refused to accept their dialysis patients before storms in the 2004 hurricane season (Hyer et al. 2009).

Hospitals remained open during both Hurricane Katrina and Hurricane Sandy. During Hurricane Katrina, eleven hospitals in the New Orleans metropolitan area remained open, sheltering over 7,600 staff members and their families in addition to 1,749 patients. The hospitals that received the most publicity during and after the hurricane were Charity Hospital, University Hospital, Tulane University Hospital, Veterans Affairs Medical Center, Lindy Boggs Medical Center, and Memorial Medical Center. These hospitals lost power and were flooded, forcing a prolonged and difficult evacuation. Fink suggests that part of the problem with the evacuation of Lindy Boggs and Memorial, even though they had resources that other hospitals, such as the VA, did not, was with the implementation of the triage system, which was covered more extensively in chapter 7, "The Expected Dead." Lindy Boggs and Memorial, owned by Tenet, both implemented a reverse triage system that deprioritized the sickest and most vulnerable for evacuation (Fink 2013).

COMMUNITY-DWELLING ELDERS

As described in chapter 6, most elders, even those with a diagnosis of Alzheimer's disease, live in the community rather than in nursing homes (Callahan et al. 2012). Even people with Alzheimer's disease tend to live and die in their own homes, rather than at a skilled nursing facility. In my own research, most caregivers were only marginally aware of when their home had been built, whether it was constructed of more wind resistant cinder blocks or other materials, or if they were living in a flood zone (Christensen 2012). This means that emergency efforts ought to be focused on identifying and educating elders living in the community before a disaster strikes. Elders have unique challenges when preparing for and responding to hurricanes, which need to be considered by emergency management and public health professionals.

A SYSTEM THAT FUNCTIONS: WEST PALM BEACH SPECIAL NEEDS SHELTERS

Bernice is in her forties and suffers from liver failure. She requires dialysis on a weekly basis to clean the toxins from her blood that her liver can no longer process. Bernice is also the primary caregiver for her mother, Jean, who lives with her. Jean has trouble walking, is unable to prepare her own food, or bathe herself. Each day, Bernice helps her mother use the bathroom, assists her with getting dressed, and then makes her breakfast. She then assists Jean with her nebulizer, which, when plugged in, turns liquid medication into a mist that keeps Jean's lungs open so she can breathe.

They live in a small home on the edge of Lake Okeechobee, Florida. Lake Okeechobee is a large but shallow lake that yields rich, dark soil called "muck." This muck has made for excellent farming in Florida's warm climate, especially for sugar cane (Hollander 2008). However, Lake Okeechobee is also the second most vulnerable area to hurricane impact, right behind the city of New Orleans (Leatherman, Zhang, and Xiao 2007). If this lake were to be directly hit by a hurricane, the storm surge would essentially pick up the lake and dump it on the surrounding inhabitants. Most of the towns surrounding this lake are rural and not very wealthy; this is a poor farming area that lacks many resources. There is, however, a bus that Bernice uses to get to her doctor's appointments because she does not own a car. That same bus takes Jean to adult day care three times a week, where she can socialize and participate in activities. This gives Bernice time to take care of the home, walk to the grocery store, and go to her dialysis appointments.

Since both Bernice and Jean have "special needs" that could be life threatening if they lost power for prolonged periods of time, they both qualify for the county's special needs shelter program. Special needs shelters are run parallel to the "regular" emergency shelter system ("Special Needs Shelter Program" 2017). According to the website of the Florida Department of Health,

> A Special Needs Shelter (SpNS) is a place to go when there is no other sheltering option. Shelters may be activated during an emergency event to provide mass care for people who cannot safely remain in their home. Special needs shelters are designed to meet the needs of persons who require assistance that exceeds services provided at a general population shelter. Special needs shelters are intended to provide, to the extent possible under emergency conditions, an environment that can sustain an individual's level of health.
>
> The Florida Department of Health, Bureau of Preparedness and Response administers a statewide Special Needs Shelter Program to assist local communities in meeting the needs of special medical and vulnerable populations. ("Special Needs Shelter Program" 2017)

With her doctor's help, Bernice registers her mother and herself for the special needs shelter every year before June 1 (the official start of hurricane season). When she registers, the public transportation office is notified that Bernice and her mother will need to be picked up and transported to the special needs shelter in advance of a storm. In 2004, they were picked up and transported to the special needs shelter three times, for Hurricane Charley, Hurricane Frances, and Hurricane Jeanne. In 2005, they were transported twice, for Hurricane Katrina and Hurricane Wilma.

At the special needs shelter, Bernice told me that though there were nurses on staff at the shelter, "I basically took care of mom in the shelter. I bathed her . . . gave her sponge baths. They changed the bedding, but I did her medications." She said she especially remembered Hurricane Wilma because of how long it was before she and Jean could return home.

After Wilma, we were still in the shelter for a week because the power was still not on at home. They aren't supposed to let you leave the shelter until the area where you live has been cleared. We couldn't go back without electricity because of mom's nebulizer. . . . The power was out at our place for over three weeks. After a week, they had discharged a lot of people out of the shelter but we couldn't go home. We were transferred out of the shelter and into a nursing home. I am considered special needs too, so they admitted me too. They treated us like patients at the nursing home. I was transported to my dialysis treatments across town three days a week.

When Hurricane Isaac threatened in 2011, Bernice and Jean returned to the special needs shelter. Bernice did not want to risk the storm turning and the bus being unable to transport them to the shelter, which was over twenty-five miles away.

In 2012, Hurricane Sandy swung close to the Florida shore, and the storm bands whipped at the coastal cities. Again, Bernice and Jean were transported to the shelter. Since her mother had been diagnosed with dementia in 2010, Bernice started keeping a disaster kit that she brought with her to the special needs shelter.

Bernice and her mother provide an example of a successful implementation of "the system." Bernice and her mother demonstrated several factors that would have made them especially vulnerable to hurricanes. They both had medical needs. They did not have access to a car. They lived in a rural, impoverished area where the dikes that held back Lake Okeechobee were under repair. They lived in public housing, which did not provide hurricane shutters. They did not have much income and their social supports were limited. But the services needed to protect Bernice were available, she knew about them, and worked to access them.

With the help of a social worker, Bernice learned about the county's special needs shelter program. She understood the risk that she and her mother faced should they try to weather the storm alone in their unsafe dwelling, so she acted to utilize the services available. She worked with her doctor to ensure they had registered with the county as needing the special needs shelter. The county even arranged for a bus to pick Bernice and her mother up before any storm. Bernice knew what she needed to do to keep her mother comfortable in the shelter. Fortunately, there was never a direct hit; had there been, it is likely that Bernice and her mother would have been safer in the shelter than they would have been in their home.

I tried reaching out to Bernice in 2018 to see how she and her family fared during Hurricane Irma. The phone number I had for her no longer worked. I eventually reached her son, who told me his grandmother, Jean, had passed over a year before the call (not of hurricane-related causes). While Bernice herself likely still required ongoing dialysis treatments, her role as caregiver for a parent had ended.

Likewise, across the state in a different county, my neighbors Liz and John lost their father-in-law, Dan (see chapter 7), five months after Hurricane Irma. They were thankful, though, that they and their children were able to spend time with their grandfather before he died. They are grateful, too, that they were lucky not to have tragically lost him to drowning in their home during the storm because they could not get into a special needs shelter. He died peacefully.

CRACKS IN THE SYSTEM

During Hurricane Irma, I learned that there were fewer trained American Red Cross volunteers running fewer shelters in Florida. Due to more accurate flood maps, the Red Cross had fewer spaces that met their safety standards. The county, however, continued to run shelters in schools located in zones the Red Cross would not. The result was understaffed and undertrained volunteers attempting to run shelters in schools. The rapid shifting of Hurricane Irma meant that more people were attempting to use shelters, and more were opened within 24 hours of the storm hitting. The schools did not have adequate supplies, such as toilet paper, which created unsanitary conditions.

The conditions in shelters have been difficult to assess. While after the storm there were stories appearing on social media describing the conditions of the schools that served as shelters, they were taken down within days. I conducted informal interviews with anyone I met after the storm and the stories I heard were alarming. One woman, Jen, in her thirties, went to a high school for shelter during Hurricane Irma. She had her fifteen-month-old son with her. As she was registering, there were older people sitting on the floor in the lobby. She was told they were "getting a place ready for them" because they had special needs, like requiring oxygen tanks. A group of people wearing maroon uniforms arrived, bringing elderly individuals in wheelchairs and walkers. This detail suggests they worked at a long-term care facility, but I have not been able to confirm this. One man was being pushed in a wheelchair and tried to say hi to Jen's son, but the caregiver yelled at him and wheeled him away. The people in uniform did not stay once the people they brought were registered. Jen reported that the people were on the floor for approximately twenty hours before they were placed. She heard them asking repeatedly when they would get a bed. During the storm, the school lost power and it was hot. There was no running water. The shelter ran out of food by the second day. So the volunteers just passed out water. While water is essential, this situation reflects hastily planned shelters. The government has avoided full responsibility in locating shelters, training volunteers, or stocking food and water in case of emergency by relying on the American Red Cross, a nongovernmental agency, largely run by volunteers. When they deemed shelters too risky to open, the responsibility of sheltering citizens fell back to the local governments.

SUMMARY

As discussed in chapter 8, the built environment, especially in large coastal cities, can amplify vulnerability to hurricanes. Nursing homes and assisted living facilities (ALFs) are part of the built environment. People who reside in skilled nursing facilities are largely dependent on staff to make the best decisions possible about their health care needs before, during, and after a storm. There are federal guidelines that govern disaster plans for skilled nursing facilities and there are many resources available to assist administrators and staff in making those decisions, including whether to evacuate a facility or shelter in place. Assisted living facilities, while required to have a policy on disaster planning, can vary widely in provisions and structures, some requiring residents to leave the premises during a storm. People with medical needs living in the community usually have the option of staying in county-run special needs shelters, though there are multiple restrictions on who can use them. Most require signing up for the shelter, with the help of a doctor, well before the beginning of hurricane season. Facilities that provide essential medical services, including skilled nursing facilities, must be incorporated into essential disaster planning services. The failure of critical infrastructure, such as medical facilities, can contribute to loss of life, especially for vulnerable elders. There are multiple examples of successful disaster preparedness response for elders with medical needs in the community that can serve as models for other services. Some of these will be addressed in chapter 10.

Chapter Ten

Connections and Potential Solutions

WORLDVIEW AND ORIGIN STORIES

In 1988, Bill Moyers conducted several interviews with mythologist Joseph Campbell (Campbell and Moyers 1988). At the beginning of their fifth interview, exploring how our origin stories influence society and shape our worldviews, Moyers opened with the words of Chief Seattle (1852):

> The President in Washington sends word that he wishes to buy our land. But how can you buy or sell the sky, the land? The idea is strange to us. Every part of this earth is sacred to my people. Every shining pine needle, every sandy shore, every mist in the dark woods, every meadow, all are holy in the memory and experience of my people. We're part of the earth and it is part of us. The perfumed flowers are our sisters. The bear, the deer, the great eagle, these are our brothers. Each ghostly reflection in the clear water of the lakes tells of events and memories in the life of my people. The water's murmur is the voice of my father's father; the rivers are our brothers. They carry our canoes and feed our children. If we sell you our land, remember that the air is precious to us, that the air shares its spirit with all the life it supports. The wind that gave our grandfather his first breath also receives his last sigh. This we know: the earth does not belong to man. Man belongs to the earth. All things are connected, like the blood that unites us all. Man did not weave the web of life, he is merely a strand in it. Whatever he does to the web, he does to himself.

Moyers used these words to describe how origin stories also shifted when humans moved away from hunter-gatherer societies and into more sedentary, agricultural or agrarian societies.

Sacred places: Delphi, Machu Picchu, Stonehenge, Jerusalem. We recognize these as places where societies came together to express their spiritual concerns. But for some very early societies, as Joseph Campbell points out in his *Historical Atlas of World Mythology*, the whole earth was a sacred place, whether living on the wide plains under the great dome of the open sky, or in dense forest under a canopy of trees, our ancestors saw the sacred in everything around them. The voices of the gods spoke from the wind and thunder, and the spirit of God flowed in every mountain stream. It was a geography not of city and nation-states, but of sacred places, the realm of the mythic imagination.

As our ancestors turned from hunting to planting, the stories they told to interpret the mysteries of life changed, too. Now the seed instead of the animal became the symbol of life, death, and resurrection. The plant died, was buried, and its seed born again. To spiritual visionaries this image reveals a divine truth as well as a principle of life itself. From death comes life; from sacrifice, bliss.

In many ways, Moyers and Campbell are giving a synopsis of the study of anthropology. In an introduction to anthropology course, instructors cover all subfields of anthropology: biological, cultural, linguistic, archaeology, and sometimes, applied anthropology. It traces the existence of the genus *Homo*, how they related to their world, how they used culture to adapt, how they made meaning (Haviland et al. 2014). They consider all other primates that existed in the past, those that went extinct, and those few that continue to exist today. In the span of a semester or a quarter term, students are exposed to a wide range of concepts that help them understand the human condition. In biological anthropology, students learn about genetics and the forces of micro and macro evolution and biocultural connections. In cultural anthropology, students learn about human diversity, how societies are grouped by age and gender, economic systems, subsistence patterns, politics of power and violence, spirituality, religion, and the supernatural. In linguistics, communication, meaning, symbolism, and signaling create affiliations with groups. In archaeology, students study the recovery of human and material remains, using those remains to reconstruct the ecology, built environment, social structures, and values of a society. Archaeology can help us understand both our biological and cultural adaptations to environmental and social pressures of the past.

SCIENCE, SKEPTICISM, AND ANTISCIENCE SENTIMENTS

In the United States, there are strong antiscience trends on both the far left and far right of the political spectrum. Both are skeptical of government intervention, including public health movements. A rejection of vaccinations is one issue where there is antiscience overlap between the political extremes. There is historical basis for some of this skepticism: the government has been involved in flawed and deeply unethical research, such as the Tuskegee syphilis study. The Tuskegee syphilis study used unwitting African American participants to learn about the natural progression of the disease. The doctors even blocked at least fifty of their participants from receiving treatment that could have cured them (Thomas and Quinn 1991). Historical context such as this can help explain hesitation to accept research findings or public health assistance from the government. History has shown that a certain level of distrust is warranted.

On the religious right, the antiscience stance is closely tied with an insistence on a literal interpretation of the Bible, especially the origin story presented in the book of Genesis. Genesis presents an omnipotent God speaking the world into existence over the course of six days (and resting on the seventh) and giving humans literal dominion over plants and animals. Among people who adhere to a literal interpretation, Earth is widely believed to be six thousand years old (Ham 1998). Scientists are viewed with skepticism because they present explanatory models that contrast with the literal interpretation of the Bible on which this belief system is built. Unfortunately, literal interpretations of the Bible correlate with lower levels of environmental concern, reinforcing the suggestion made by Campbell and Moyers in 1988 (Schultz, Zelezny, and Dalrymple 2000; Greeley 1993; Smith and Leiserowitz 2013; Morrison, Duncan, and Parton 2015).

Anthropology instructors have an opportunity to witness the struggle between the scientific approach and the desire to adhere to a religious framework in their classrooms. Though science and religion need not be mutually exclusive, they are often approached as if they are in conservative theological teachings and, conversely, by many scientists. This conflict shows itself as we discuss human ancestors and the genetic and physiological resemblance to other primates and the concept of evolution. It is sometimes interpreted by conservative Christians as a fundamental assault on their person. While the scientific process is the product of human endeavors, it seeks to minimize false pattern recognition and cultural biases as one explains the world. The conservative Christian tradition asks practitioners to take the word of the Bible on faith, regardless of observations presented via the scientific process.

When it comes to the relationship between humans, their environment, and climate change, not only does the book of Genesis state that God created the world in seven days, it gives humans dominion over all plants and animals. It places them above all other living things (though below God). This framework, as noted by Campbell, provides an orientation toward consumption and a fear or disregard for nature (though it is not always interpreted this way, which will be discussed below).

Campbell and Moyers famously pointed out that Abrahamic orientations see God as separate from nature.

> Now, in the other mythologies, one puts oneself in accord with the world. If the world is a mixture of good and evil, you do not put yourself in accord with it. You identify with the good and you fight against the evil, and this is a religious system which belongs to the Near East, following Zarathustra's time. It's in the biblical tradition, all the way, in Christianity and in Islam as well. This business of not being with nature, and we speak with sort of derogation of "the nature religions." You see, with that fall in the garden, nature was regarded as corrupt. There's a myth for you that corrupts the whole world for us. And every spontaneous act is sinful, because nature is corrupt and has to be corrected, must not be yielded to. You get a totally different civilization, a totally different way of living according to your myth as to whether nature is fallen or whether nature is itself a manifestation of divinity, and the spirit being the revelation of the divinity that's inherent in nature. (Campbell and Moyers 1988)

How might this orientation toward the world shape economic policies, environmental preservation, and development? Humans like to form in-groups and out-groups, associating with others who are similar. Signaling their belonging to a group can range from using different languages or speech patterns, clothing styles, type of vehicle driven, to the stories that one "believes."

In the United States, the religious right is tied to conservative social and economic policies: traditional gender roles, deregulating markets, removing regulations on environmental protections, and expanding consumption of fossil fuels.

Scientists know that humans are causing unprecedented climate change, which is fueling increasingly destructive, weather-related events. Scientists also know what we need to do to stop it: reduce our reliance on fossil fuels and shift our investments to renewable energies, and plan our communities in a more efficient way that reduces reliance on cars and makes it easier for people of all ages to remain mobile and productive. There are ideological barriers to these solutions, which must be recognized and addressed, or they are unlikely to be changed.

Cultural anthropologists work to understand those they study to be able to explain the world as the people they study view it. Applied anthropologists often work as cultural brokers to translate that understanding into advocacy. As scientists ourselves, it can be frustrating to work with and respond to people in our own society who reject science, especially at the cost of environmental stability. It can perhaps be useful to consider the topics of evolution and climate change as an opportunity to practice cultural relativism.

UNDERSTANDING (DIS)BELIEF

Humans are social animals. We need each other. Despite the rather individualistic slant of modern Western society, we tend to identify with certain groups, whether they be sports teams, hometown, nation of origin, profession, or religious affiliation. We signal identification with those groups in multiple ways, sometimes through the type of car we drive, sometimes by the type of bumper sticker we put on that car. In more extreme cultural initiations, belief systems are ascribed to and signaled through ritual displays (Watson-Jones and Legare 2016). This process was documented by Durkheim, who described "ritual as strengthening group cohesion" (Watson-Jones and Legare 2016, 42).

A "good Christian" believes one thing, such as the divine creation of the earth and humans, and rejects another, like the concept of evolution. The implicit belief that humans have dominion over the earth, or the belief that God will take care of the problem seeps into the political rejection of climate change. It becomes a signal of belonging. This signal can be the public rejection of a body of scientific evidence, whether by openly challenging a professor, making statements on social media, or having a "Jesus Fish" on one's car. Conversely, placing a "Jesus Fish" that has a set of legs on one's car signals a belief in evolution.

Ignorance is not always a gap in knowledge: "Ignorance in the realm of science is typically depicted as a gap in knowledge: something that we do not (yet) know. But the condition of not knowing is not (always) as simple as that" (Tuana 2006). It takes a great amount of effort to reject a body of knowledge and to preserve group fidelity. The world of comedy provided an example of this: Samantha Bee devoted an episode of her show, *Full Frontal with Samantha Bee*, to the issue of climate change (Harkin 2017). One of her correspondents, Harkin, went to Tangier Island. Harkin narrates, "A tiny speck in Chesapeake Bay, Tangier is home to a small and very religious community of hardy crabbers." The camera shows a large poster of a giant Jesus Fish with the words "we believe" outside a home as she sails by with the mayor, James Eskridge. Harkin continues, "Tragically, Tangier is rapidly disappearing into the Chesapeake because of sea level rise." Though the residents of the island see that the land is disappearing below the sea and that their lawns are becoming a salt-water swamp, they blame the phenomenon on erosion. Interestingly, the only people interviewed are white men over the age of fifty. Most of those interviewed, including the mayor, identify as evangelical Christians. A Jesus Fish is painted on the helm of his boat (as is a Star of David). Mayor Eskridge insists that "erosion, not sea level rise" is what is causing the island to be engulfed by the surrounding ocean. Harkin meets with several men from the community where she discusses climate change. One of those men, George, an older white man, tells Harkin that climate change is "the biggest hoax there ever was." They also ask Harkin if she believes in evolution, phrasing it as, "Do you think that I evolved from an ape?" (which, anthropologists would point out, is not an accurate depiction of how evolution works). When Harkin says she does believe in evolution, they respond, "We'll put you on our prayer list." Harkin intentionally sought out this group of people, who have much to lose from denying climate change.

Maureen Coyle, a professor at the University of Toronto, seeks to work through her own consternation at why people might reject the science behind climate change, even if it is directly affecting them. Coyle, like myself, is particularly interested in how climate change affects older populations in an aging world. She wonders why people who have much to lose by denying climate change and little to gain (unlike those who own oil companies) would continue to deny climate change. The men in the *Full Frontal* episode were prime examples of this group.

In her article, Coyle writes, "Fifty years after the emergence of warnings over the effects of the environmental impacts of industrialization and other conditions of a planet subjugated by humans, we are still entertaining discussions about the existence of the phenomena of climate change" (2015, 76).

The word "subjugated" echoes the Western idea that humans have dominion over the world around them.

While it is easier to understand why people with a vested interest in fossil fuels (the Koch brothers) or land development (Bush and Trump families) might deny climate change, it is more difficult and concerning when a person with little to gain and much to lose embraces ignorance:

> Do people who decry discussions of climate change benefit in some way—directly or indirectly—from these industries? Or are they fearful that if they need to take climate change seriously, they will be required to give up something that has a negative impact on them; something which they, as Erving Goffman might suggest, draw upon to form their presentation of self—something like a job, for example, or a car—or other aspects of social presentation that are the means to display social and economic capital. That climate change denial exists in this context of immediate self-interest, such as is evident among some legislators, is less puzzling than that among the general populace, because the lines of self-interest are much clearer in the case of the public officials. Private citizens have more to lose by denying climate change and less to gain by denial. (Coyle 2015, 79)

To better work through the situation, Coyle applies the concept of "epistemologies of ignorance" (originally conceptualized by Tuana 2004) to understand why climate change has become a point of contention among the general population. She explains that Tuana developed the epistemologies of ignorance to explain how so little could be understood about the female reproductive system. She argues that,

> if we are to fully understand the complex practices of knowledge production and the variety of factors that account for why something is known, we must also understand the practices that account for not knowing, that is, for our lack of knowledge about a phenomenon or, in some case, an account of practices that resulted in the group unlearning what was once a realm of knowledge. (Tuana 2006)

The epistemology of ignorance is divided into six categories.

1. Knowing that we do not know, but not caring to know.
2. We do not even know that we do not know.
3. They do not want us to know.
4. Willful ignorance.

5. Ignorance produced by the construction of epistemically disadvantaged identities.
6. Loving ignorance and accepting what we cannot know.

Coyle argues that

> this taxonomy is a means of understanding ignorance, and positions that help maintain a constructed position in the face of clear evidence to the contrary, and it may be useful in understanding the resistance to action to counter climate change, not just among older adults, but also among policy makers and politicians who have been less cooperative than required to enact a halt, if not a reversal, of the damage done to the Earth and to the atmosphere. (2015, 80)

The taxonomy of ignorance has many facets, but I found some more helpful when thinking about resistance to climate change than others: (1) knowing that we do not know, but not caring to know; (2) they do not want us to know; (3) willful ignorance.

Knowing that we do not know, but not caring to know. The funding mechanisms for science are such that scientists must justify why they seek to learn something. As Tuana writes, "scientists do not aimlessly chase truth." Funders, whether public or private, determine what is worthy of study. (Tuana uses the example of male birth control, which while possible, was not deemed worthy of scientific pursuit.) Those who benefit from oil extraction or other lucrative fossil fuel–related fields or land development are perhaps more likely to ascribe to this category of ignorance. Why would they want to learn more about an endangered species if they could make money drilling or paving its habitat? It may be seen "in the same way that ignorance is a necessary cost of progress"; it is an "uninteresting detail that we will be able to iron out later (Coyle 2015, 82). Tuana argues that "this form of ignorance works to protect authority from scrutiny" (2006).

We do not even know that we do not know. This type of ignorance is found in situations in which "current interests or knowledge block such knowledge, like, 'things have always been this way'" (Tuana 2006, 6, as quoted in Coyle 2015). This is like an unconscious bias that is difficult to recognize because we are so steeped in a way of living.

They do not want us to know. This is when certain types of knowledge are deemed "too dangerous" for some to have. "In this category I place topics or technologies that are known, but are kept secret, where selected groups of people are purposely kept ignorant." Concerns for profit are often in this realm. Tuana uses the example of the danger of smoking tobacco, and the side effects of the original contraceptives. As mentioned in chapter 2, the same architects of the confusion about the harms of tobacco have also been instrumental in obscuring the anthropogenic factors in climate change (Oreskes and Conway 2010a; Hevesi 2008). When development contracts are kept secret, access to information can be limited. Information on who is directly benefiting from drilling in national parks, for example, might not be immediately clear if not for the work of investigative journalists. The public is intentionally kept in ignorance.

Willful ignorance. Here, Tuana uses Marilyn Frye's concept of "ignorance" as it was applied to racism, "positions of privilege in oppressive contexts such as racism exhibit a 'determined ignorance' of the lives and histories of those deemed 'inferior.' . . . Ignorance is not passive, but to begin to appreciate this, one need only hear the active verb 'to ignore' in the word 'ignorance'" (Frye 1983, 119, as cited in Tuana 2006). Coyle connects willful ignorance with climate change in this way: "Failure to understand that the widespread use of fossil fuels is harmful, or that unbridled use of plastics and other chemicals, or failure to consider waste disposal is an 'active production and preservation of ignorance'" (Tuana 2006, 10).The prevalence of research showing the correlation between far right (usually white) evangelical Christians and what is potentially willful ignorance suggests in-group signals.

BRIDGING THE DIVIDE

Harkin's *Full Frontal* segment, in which she spent time on Tangier Island, was not meant to poke fun at willful ignorance, but to find a better way to discuss climate change in a community resistant to the idea. Harkin sits in the kitchen area with the small group of residents of Tangier Island (2017). To convince the residents that their island was disappearing because of sea level rise, related to climate change, she offered to bring Al Gore to speak to them, to which one man responded: "We don't want that trash here. Make sure you put that statement on that camera. I don't want you, Al Gore!"

Harkin explains through narration that she had consulted experts before coming to Tangier Island, "I prepared by speaking to Katharine Hayhoe." The camera cuts to Dr. Katharine Hayhoe as she gives a lecture on climate change and religion: "God gave us responsibility over our planet." On the screen behind her are the words "Let us make human beings in our image, make them reflecting our nature so they can be responsible for every living thing that moves on the face of Earth." Hayhoe makes the argument that "just saying, oh, God will take care of it or it doesn't matter is actually a profoundly un-Christian perspective. In the Bible it says, 'God will destroy those who destroy the Earth.'" She recommends that Harkin first listen: "The first way to connect is to listen. Rather than coming in saying, 'I know! I am going to tell you, you listen to me,' the place to start is by sharing from the heart. What is it that we have in common?" (Which Harkin paraphrases as: "So don't start the conversation by being a dick.") The camera cuts to Harkin speaking with the Tangier Island mayor, James Eskridge, "I love crabs. I'm assuming you like crabs?" After some other attempts at finding common ground, the camera cuts back to Harkin with Dr. Hayhoe, "And then you ask them for their stories. Have you noticed anything changing? Ask them." Harkin does, indeed, ask the group of older men: "Has the weather changed since you were a little boy?" They admit it has changed but explain that it probably just goes through cycles.

Harkin: "Do you believe that the ice is melting in the Arctic?"

George: "Yeah, it is. But I don't worry about that."

Harkin: "Even when your feet are getting wet on your front lawn?"

The man, George, explained that once the rapture happens, no one will have to worry about the melting ice caps. Harkin, using Hayhoe's strategy, says: "Let me throw this out there and we'll let it land. We don't even have to discuss it. What if climate scientists are actually doing God's work?" After a thoughtful silence, the men agreed, that yes, God could be working through climate scientists, who aim to protect the environment. However, they refuse to acknowledge that something called "climate change" is happening.

While intended to bring humor to a difficult subject, this segment draws upon research. Hayhoe's methods have been proven (Webb and Hayhoe 2017). What is more, the ethos of this method, based in listening and learning, is also at the heart of most qualitative research, including ethnography, employed by anthropologists and sociologists.

Rejection of these concepts, though based on numerous verifiable facts, can be a demonstration of faith. Hayhoe has an advantage because, as a Christian herself, she is demonstrating how the Bible can make room for better care for the environment. She can signal her identification with the group in other ways, through her knowledge of scripture and her understanding of what is important to the group.

It is important to note that it is not just white, evangelical Christians who resist the concept of climate change; many who distrust "the system" may also reject it. Elders themselves, who have lived a lifetime of experiences and have seen the experts provide predictions that have not come to bear, may be "natural skeptics" (Moody 2015). Examination of climate change denial can provide guidance for the development of a better counternarrative. There are many things that individuals can do to reduce their own impact, and specific policies they can advocate for at the local, state, and national level.

SUGGESTIONS AND SOLUTIONS FOR CHANGE AT ALL LEVELS

Once one can communicate about the need for addressing climate change, perhaps people will be more willing to make small shifts in their way of living. Living in a healthy, responsible way can be expensive. When people are working minimum-wage jobs, worrying about getting food on the table, it will be more difficult to prioritize recycling. Nonetheless, many people are looking for small ways to be socially and environmentally responsible. These suggestions are made in good faith, recognizing that they will not be relevant or practical for all people.

Individual-Level Lifestyle Choices

1. Reduce, reuse, recycle.

    a. Use reusable shopping bags. Plastics are derived from fossil fuels and are not biodegradable.
    b. Use reusable water bottles rather than plastic bottles and coffee cups whenever possible.
    c. Avoid single-serve coffee pods that include the plastic cup casing. There are styles available that just have the filter without the plastic cup casing. If there is more than one coffee drinker in the household, avoid coffee pods entirely. Use a standard coffee machine. Consider switching to black tea, which uses less water to grow.
    d. Reduce meat and animal products to reduce demand for factory farming (a large producer of methane).

2. Reduce energy consumption.

    a. Replace standard lightbulbs with LED lights.
    b. Turn out lights when leaving.
    c. Turn down AC and heat when leaving the house.

3. Push for zoning requirements that allow for green roofs and lighter-colored roofing materials (which can reflect the sun and reduce the heat island effect).
4. Use semipermeable bricks for driveway construction.
5. If living in a house with a yard, plant trees to reduce ambient temperature.
6. Lobby for public transportation. When available, use public transportation.
7. Lobby for sidewalks and bike lanes to make it safer to travel without a car.
8. Choose to live in high-density housing. Apartment buildings and condos allow more people to live in less space. Though perhaps less prestigious, it is a better use of land than a suburban home.
9. Grow your own foods, or buy local, if possible, thereby reducing the need to transport produce from far away. It can also reduce the demand for plastic packaging.
10. Be skeptical of politicians who come from a land development or fossil fuel development background. They are likely to be torn between constituent desires for environmental preservation and the practices that have made them wealthy. While it is possible that their interests will remain with constituents, be vigilant.
11. Be aware of the recent history of segregation in the United States and how it might contribute to environmental racism. When possible, lend your voice to support those who have been historically marginalized.

Individual-Level Practices during Heat Waves or without Electricity after Storms

1. Put a wet washcloth on your neck. If a battery-powered fan is available, the combination can help cool the body.
2. Put supplements that have electrolytes (such as Emergen-C) or Nuun tablets in emergency kits.

3. Wash juice and ice tea bottles, fill with tap water, and store in the house.
4. Include a LifeStraw filter or iodine tablets in a disaster kit to purify water (in case of boil-water orders).
5. Invest in a battery-powered fan to help circulate air. A hybrid model might be best, because it can remain useful when plugged in when power is available.
6. Refill medications before the storm.

Recommendations at the County/City Level

1. Consider banning plastic bags. Adopt compostable plastics for fast food. Ensure facilities are available that can compost those plastics (most must be composted by a special process, not in one's own backyard compost). Provide education about this process.
2. Provide access to safe modes of transportation beyond a personal vehicle. Make and enforce laws that protect pedestrians. Require developers to include sidewalks in their plans. Require them to replace a tree for each tree that is removed for development. Calculate the permeable and impermeable materials used. Allow and provide incentives for green roofs and encourage lighter-colored roofing materials (Gonzalez 2010; Stone 2012).
3. Plan better for disasters. Ensure safe locations for emergency shelters. If they do not exist, prioritize funding to build them. Provide adequate training for staff.
4. Lieutenant General Honoré, who commanded Joint Task Force Katrina, recommended that more people volunteer with the American Red Cross so that the local community can be better prepared when disaster strikes. He specifically suggested that more colleges and universities start Red Cross Clubs (personal communication, March 24, 2018).

   a. I recommend incorporating training for volunteers to better serve elderly individuals in emergency shelter situations. For example, a training unit on how to respond to someone who might have dementia. Dementia related behaviors can be exacerbated with a change in location, making evacuation to shelters more challenging for volunteers, caregivers, and the person with the disease.

5. Access to pet-friendly emergency shelters is critical to ensure evacuation, especially for older adults (Douglas 2017).

During Emergencies: Special Needs Shelters

1. Designating shelters and training: the county needs better planning and training to accommodate elders. They need to be prepared for assisted living facilities or informal caregivers to "dump" people at shelters.
2. Flood zones. If there are not adequate spaces, they need to be built with the use of shelters in mind.
3. Create safe evacuation spaces.
4. Be prepared for pets, even if specifically not allowed (Douglas 2017).

Nursing Homes/Assisted Living Facilities/Hospitals

1. Many hospitals and nursing homes have emergency backup power located at lower levels, such as basements. Basements are prone to flooding during storms that can cause power failures (Hyer et al. 2009).
2. Allow staff families to shelter in the facility so that staff loyalties are not divided. Retrain on recognizing signs of heat stroke annually (Hyer et al. 2009).
3. Critically assess the utility and philosophies behind triage and reverse triage (Fink 2013). Train staff for extreme emergency situations and how to implement triage in the most ethical way possible.
4. Recognize nursing homes as critical infrastructure and prioritize for power restoration (Hyer et al. 2009).

State-Level Suggestions

1. Update building codes. Consider providing grants to update older homes (outside flood zones).
2. Standardize regulations for special needs shelters (Christensen 2012).
3. Support community-based long-term care, but also adequately fund Medicaid-funded nursing home beds (Christensen 2012).

Federal-Level Recommendations

1. Monitor trade policies. Recycling plastic has been exported to China, but they are beginning to refuse it (Profita and Burns 2017). Taiwan has proposed banning all plastics by 2030 (Rose 2018).
2. End *Citizens United*. Large companies and affluent individuals have long held disproportionate power in policy. But a new Supreme Court ruling, *Citizens United*, decided in 2010, has exacerbated the issue and diminished the voice of citizens. It is allowing companies to frame public health policy issues rather than science-based facts about health risks (Wiist 2011; Lima and Galea 2018).
3. Recognize that continued dependence on fossil fuels is a security threat. Rather than focusing on domestic extraction, shift focus to sustainable energy sources (Scott 2008; Singer 2010).

    a. Supplement installation of solar panels at the household and business level to make it accessible for more people.

4. Provide hurricane shutters in hurricane-prone areas to protect those who require HUD housing. Hurricane shutters would also protect the government's own assets (the physical structure) (Christensen 2012).

At the International Level

Policy for reducing emissions can be addressed at the international level (e.g., the Kyoto Protocol), the federal level (e.g., by the US government), as well as at the state, county, or municipal level. Most of the strategies at the international, federal, and state levels focus less on the built environment and more on regulating emissions of industry through other means, such as cap-and-trade, command-and-control, or carbon taxes.

MARKET-BASED INSTRUMENTS AND CARBON REDUCTION TECHNOLOGIES

Cap-and-trade is a type of "polluter pays" agreement. Under a cap-and-trade program, certain allowances are allocated to polluters; companies might be given "permits" for each of the different gases they emit (Pearce and Ahn 2017). They can obtain these permits from the initial allocation from the government or by trading between companies. The purpose of this strategy is to provide economic incentives for companies to reduce emissions. Companies that can reduce their emissions can then sell their "permits" to other companies whose production process emits more pollutants. This process has been successful in reducing sulfur dioxide (SO_2) emissions (the cause of acid rain), along with command-and-control schemes.

Command-and-control was one of the earliest forms of emissions control in the United States and was effective in reducing SO_2. Technology was developed to "scrub" the sulfur dioxide out of emissions (by changing the combustion process of coal) (Hsu 2011). Coal-fired power plants were then required ("commanded") to install the sulfur dioxide reduction technology to control emissions. Up to 90 percent of the sulfur dioxide emissions were removed from the coal-burning process. This process, while effective, does not reduce the reliance on coal. Likewise, if reliable technology were to be developed to remove CO_2 from the combustion of gasoline, it would not reduce the reliance on fossil fuels themselves.

Gonzalez argues that policies supporting technological solutions to CO_2 emissions fail to address the wider problems underlying the cause of the US dependency on fossil fuels and that the focus should be on the built environment and land use. He further argues that environmental groups should cease to lobby politicians directly because politicians are only interested in solutions that are in line with neoliberal philosophy and policy, such as relying on the development of and investment in CO_2-reducing technologies. He encourages environmental groups to focus their efforts on educating the public on the underlying conditions of urban sprawl. He cites John Dryzek, a democratic theorist, who argues that "groups that critique the status quo can only participate in the policy making process to the extent that the groups' goals are consistent with the objective of the state" (1996, 479, as cited in Gonzalez 2010, 92). Gonzalez argues that this is true of the environmental groups (e.g., Sierra Club, Natural Resources Defense Council) that are active in the formulation of the federal government's climate change regime in that they are doing very little to address urban sprawl and automobile dependency. Their favored solutions are in line with the status quo, namely, to emphasize technology and alternative fuels. He argues that environmental groups are being symbolically included in the democratic policy-making process to help quell potential dissent. It gives the public the impression that real change is taking place and environmental protection policy is taking place, when in fact they are not. While Gonzalez makes some excellent points, his proposed solutions are questionable. While advocating for environmental groups to diversify their approaches and allocating more time and funds to community education and urban sprawl is essential, environmental groups should not drop their lobbying efforts within the political arena because a multipronged approach is needed to address complex sociopolitical issues such as these. We must both educate the public (find ways to speak to people resistant to the reality of climate change) *and* lobby local and state government to encourage public transportation and environmentally friendly development. Ignoring the policy and legislative component is dangerous. Lobbying to overturn *Citizens United* (argued in 2009), which has given disproportionate power to corporations rather than citizens, must be aggressively pursued if we are to achieve environmental justice (Lima and Galea 2018; Wiist 2011).

REDUCING RELIANCE ON CARS AND REDUCING THE HEAT ISLAND EFFECT

Stone also expresses concern about the failure of international policies to stem CO_2 emissions associated with climate change (2012). The focus of his concern is on the extreme heat events that take place in large metropolitan areas; like Gonzalez, he sees localized urban planning as a possible local solution to climate change. Stone, however, advocates for "replace a tree" programs in suburban areas (when a tree is removed to make room for development, developers are held responsible for planting a tree in its place). In more centralized urban areas, he suggests utilizing green roofs, such as planting gardens on the roofs of both residential and government buildings.

Mitigation at the city planning level includes the creation of more parks and green roofs and requires political buy-in from both citizens and developers. As Stone argues, green roofs and other building alternatives must not only be *allowed* by local zoning, they must be encouraged. Ultimately, effective urban planning can reduce waste-heat produced by combustion engines by providing more public transportation and pedestrian facilities, like sidewalks. Again, a multipronged approach that includes both grassroots-level community education and political lobbying might be necessary for addressing the range of barriers that can block environmentally friendly policies.

SUMMARY

An ecosyndemic is a way of explaining how a physical body exists within its social and ecological conditions and how those conditions can amplify or protect against the disease process. It incorporates the concept of syndemics, when two coexisting diseases amplify the disease processes (see chapter 2).

Chapter 1 provided a contextual story of Betsy and Joe, two people aging in a time of climate change. They provide a starting point to explore the debate about what constitutes a "disease" and what is simply part of "normal aging," which was explored in more depth in chapter 5. Normal aging is correlated with a slow decrease in some bodily functions, such as decrease in eyesight, loss of hearing, mild memory loss, and stamina. Some of this loss can be easily corrected with tools, such as glasses, hearing aids, and pen and notepad. Other correlates of aging, such as the hardening of the arteries, are less noticeable. When the decline increases to the point that a person is unable to perform daily functions (activities of daily living or ADLs) or becomes life threatening, then practitioners consider those processes to be a disease. Joe started out with what was normal memory loss, but eventually was unable to care for himself (explored further in chapter 6). His wife, Betsy, took on the role of caregiver, which is challenging under the best of circumstances and is correlated with high stress. In turn, the stress faced by caregivers can impair their own bodies' resistance to disease.

When faced with extreme weather, the underlying illnesses and diseases can become a challenge for survival (as presented in chapter 6). They can make understanding and acting on warnings more difficult or impossible. Betsy and Joe's story provides just one example of how a weather event, a hurricane, challenged their well-being and safety. They were, however, protected by their social and economic status.

We have many technologies that can mitigate aspects of normal aging, including changes in eyesight, hearing, even mobility. Some of these conditions are exacerbated by extreme heat and extreme cold, as described in chapter 5. Under controlled conditions, they need not be fatal, but without proper planning and support, they can be.

The role of caregiver is transient, as are many illnesses (Betsy lost Joe in 2012 to causes related to his Alzheimer's disease; Liz and John lost Dan in early 2018, due to his underlying respiratory conditions).

The scenario of elders and minorities bearing disproportionate mortality has become a pattern: New Orleans during Hurricane Katrina, in New York and New Jersey during Hurricane Sandy, and currently in Puerto Rico (see chapter 6). This pattern, rather than being a point of concern to be fixed, is in danger of being viewed as "the natural order of things" or "common sense."

The phenomenon of "expected loss" (Fjord 2007) was explored in depth in chapter 7.

Climate change is causing more frequent and extreme weather-related events, exacerbating normal age-related impairments and exposures to life-threatening situations. Chapter 3 explored the science behind climate change and how climate change affects human populations. To deepen this understanding, chapter 4 provided a snapshot of the archaeology of hurricanes to provide lessons from past civilizations. Our human ancestors developed in what is now east Africa and we managed to find ways to survive in all types of environments. Culture, passed on through oral tradition, was one of our most important adaptations: passing on knowledge about how to build structures, make clothing, manage fire, and read the stars and seasons. Our ancestors were mobile in a way few of our societies are now. Certainly, humans survived climatic shifts in the past. They may have even caused the destruction of their own local environments, but there is no evidence that they caused climatic shifts on a worldwide scale as we are seeing now. That has only happened since industrialization. We now have the technology to recognize what is happening and even how to slow or stop it. It is ideology that is creating a barrier to enacting solutions. Our modern settlement and subsistence patterns are threatened by the speed of our changing climate (see chapter 8, on the built environment and population geography).

There are many ways the warming trend can be mitigated. Powerful interests and people whose extreme wealth depends on sustained dependence on fossil fuels and unregulated development have worked very hard to keep solutions from becoming a reality. Underlying ideological orientations must be addressed for interventions to move forward.

References

Abatzoglou, John T., and A. Park Williams. 2016. "Impact of Anthropogenic Climate Change on Wildfire across Western US Forests." *Proceedings of the National Academy of Sciences* 113 (42): 11770–75. doi:10.1073/pnas.1607171113.

Achenbach, Joel, Abigal Hauslohner, and Patricia Sullivan. 2017. "Hurricanes Harvey and Irma Offer Sobering Lessons in the Power of Nature." *Washington Post*, September 17.

ACN Cuban News Agency. 2017. "Hurricane Irma: Severe Damages to Cuban Agriculture," September 12. http://www.cubanews.acn.cu/cuba/7287-hurricane-irma-severe-damages-to-cuban-agriculture.

Adams, Vincanne, Sharon R. Kaufman, Taslim Van Hattum, and Sandra Moody. 2011. "Aging Disaster: Mortality, Vulnerability, and Long-Term Recovery Among Katrina Survivors." *Medical Anthropology Quarterly* 30 (3): 247–70. doi:10.1080/01459740.2011.560777.Aging.

"Agencies Control Scientists' Contacts with the Media." 2004. Union of Concerned Scientists. https://www.ucsusa.org/center-for-science-and-democracy/scientific_integrity/abuses_of_science/a-to-z/agencies-control-scientists.html#.Wn9olqhKuHs.

Aleccia, JoNel. 2012. "Confusion in the Storm: Alzheimer's Patient Refused to Evacuate." NBC News, October 31. http://vitals.nbcnews.com/_news/2012/10/31/14811864-confusion-in-the-storm-alzheimers-patient-refused-to-evacuate?lite.

Allen, Patricia J. 2015. "Climate Change: A Review of Potential Health Consequences." *Primary Health Care* 25 (7): 34–40. doi:10.4172/2167-1079.1000183.

Allen, S. K., V. Barros, I. Burton, D. L. Lendrum, Omar-Dario Cardona, S. L. Cutter, O. P. Dube, et al. 2012. *Managing the Risks of Extreme Events and Disasters to Advance Climate Change Adaptation*. Edited by Christopher B. Field, Vicente Barros, Thomas F. Stocker, and Qin Dahe. Cambridge: Cambridge University Press. doi:10.1017/CBO9781139177245.

Almer, Christian, Jérémy Laurent-Lucchetti, and Manuel Oechslin. 2017. "Water Scarcity and Rioting: Disaggregated Evidence from Sub-Saharan Africa." *Journal of Environmental Economics and Management* 86 (November): 193–209. doi:10.1016/j.jeem.2017.06.002.

Altizer, Sonia, Richard S. Ostfeld, Pieter T. J. Johnson, Susan Kutz, and C. Drew Harvell. 2013. "Climate Change and Infectious Diseases: From Evidence to a Predictive Framework." *Science* 341 (6145): 514–19. http://www.ncbi.nlm.nih.gov/pubmed/23908230.

Alzheimer's Association. 2013. "Alzheimer's Disease Facts and Figures 2013." *Alzheimer's & Dementia* 9 (2). https://www.alz.org/downloads/facts_figures_2013.pdf.

———. 2017. "Alzheimer's Disease Facts and Figures 2017." *Alzheimer's & Dementia* 13: 325–73. https://www.alz.org/documents_custom/2017-facts-and-figures.pdf.

Anderegg, William R. L., James W. Prall, Jacob Harold, and Stephen H. Schneider. 2010. "Expert Credibility in Climate Change." *Proceedings of the National Academy of Sciences* 107 (27): 12107–109. doi:10.1073/pnas.1003187107.

Aud, Myra A. 2004. "Dangerous Wandering: Elopements of Older Adults with Dementia from Longterm Care Facilities." *American Journal of Alzheimer's Disease and Other Dementias.* 19:361–68.

Avenanti, Alessio, Angela Sirigu, and Salvatore M. Aglioti. 2010. "Racial Bias Reduces Empathic Sensorimotor Resonance with Other-Race Pain." *Current Biology* 20 (11): 1018–22. doi:10.1016/j.cub.2010.03.071.

Backer, Lorraine, Deana Manassaram-Baptiste, Rebecca LePrell, and Birgit Bolton. 2015. "Cyanobacteria and Algae Blooms: Review of Health and Environmental Data from the Harmful Algal Bloom-Related Illness Surveillance System (HABISS) 2007–2011." *Toxins* 7 (4):1048–64. doi:10.3390/toxins7041048.

Backer, Lorraine, and Dennis McGillicuddy. 2006. "Harmful Algal Blooms at the Interface between Coastal Oceanography and Human Health." *Oceanography* 19 (2):94–106. doi:10.5670/oceanog.2006.72.

Baer, Hans A. 2016. "Private Cars as Environmental Health Hazards: The Critical Need for Public Transit in the Era of Climate Change." In *A Companion to the Anthropology of Environmental Health*, edited by Merrill Singer, 458. Hoboken, NJ: John Wiley & Sons. doi:10.1002/9781118786949.

Baer, Hans A., and Merrill Singer. 2008. *Global Warming and the Political Ecology of Health: Emerging Crises and Systemic Solutions*. Walnut Creek, CA: Left Coast Press.

———. 2014. *The Anthropology of Climate Change: An Integrated Critical Perspective*. New York: Routledge.

Baer, Hans A., Merrill Singer, and John H. Johnsen. 1986. "Introduction to Critical Medical Anthropology." *Social Science & Medicine* 23 (2): 95–98. doi:http://dx.doi.org.ezproxy.lib.usf.edu/10.1016/0277-9536(86)90358-8.

Baptiste, Nathalie. 2017. "Here's What We Know About Global Warming and Hurricanes." *Mother Jones*, August 25. http://www.motherjones.com/environment/2017/08/heres-what-we-know-about-global-warming-and-hurricanes/.

Barbaro, Michael. 2018. "'The Daily': Hurricane Maria's Toll." *New York Times*, February 9. https://www.nytimes.com/2018/02/09/podcasts/the-daily/puerto-rico-hurricane-maria-deaths.html?smid=tw-share.

Barile, P. J. 2018. "Widespread Sewage Pollution of the Indian River Lagoon System, Florida (USA) Resolved by Spatial Analyses of Macroalgal Biogeochemistry." *Marine Pollution Bulletin* 128: 557–74.

Barnes, Jay. 2007. *Florida Hurricane History,* 2nd ed. Chapel Hill: University of North Carolina Press.

Barros, V., T. F. Stocker, D. Qin, D. J. Dokken, K. L. Ebi, M. D. Mastrandrea, K. J. Mach, S. K. Allen, and M. Tignor. 2014. "Glossary of Terms." *Scandinavian Journal of Public Health* 42 (14 suppl): 178–90. doi:10.1177/1403494813515131.

Bartlett, Jeff, Michelle Naranjo, and Jeff Plungis. 2017. "Guide to the Volkswagen Emissions Recall: An FAQ with Everything You Need to Know about the VW 'Dieselgate.'" *Consumer Reports*, October 23. https://www.consumerreports.org/cro/cars/guide-to-the-volkswagen-dieselgate-emissions-recall-.

BBC News. 2015. "Malcom Turnbull Sworn In as New Australian Prime Minister." September 15. http://www.bbc.com/news/world-australia-34253013.

———. 2017. "Trump Signs Order Undoing Obama Climate Change Policies." March 29. http://www.bbc.com/news/world-us-canada-39415631.

Beck, Ulrich. 1986. *Risk Society: Towards a New Modernity,* 2nd ed. London: Sage Publications.

Benestad, Rasmus E., Dana Nuccitelli, Stephan Lewandowsky, Katharine Hayhoe, Hans Olav Hygen, Rob van Dorland, and John Cook. 2016. "Learning from Mistakes in Climate Research." *Theoretical and Applied Climatology* 126 (3–4): 699–703. doi:10.1007/s00704-015-1597-5.

Beniston, Martin, and Henry F. Diaz. 2004. "The 2003 Heat Wave as an Example of Summers in a Greenhouse Climate? Observations and Climate Model Simulations for Basel, Switzerland." *Global and Planetary Change* 44:73–81.

Berchtold, N. C., and C. W. Cotman. 1998. "Evolution in the Conceptualization of Dementia and Alzheimer's Disease: Greco-Roman Period to the 1960s." *Neurobiology of Aging* 19 (3): 173–89. doi:10.1016/S0197-4580(98)00052-9.

Berg, Robbie. 2013. "Tropical Cyclone Report: Hurricane Isaac." *National Hurricane Center Tropical Cyclone Report.* http://www.nhc.noaa.gov/data/tcr/AL092012_Isaac.pdf.

Berkman, Paul Arthur, and Alexander N. Vylegzhanin, eds. 2013. *Environmental Security in the Arctic Ocean.* NATO Science for Peace and Security Series C: Environmental Security. Dordrecht: Springer Netherlands. doi:10.1007/978-94-007-4713-5.

Betsill, Michele M. 2017. "Trump's Paris Withdrawal and the Reconfiguration of Global Climate Change Governance." *Chinese Journal of Population Resources and Environment* 15 (3): 189–91, July 3. doi:10.1080/10042857.2017.1343908.

Beven, John L. 2004. "Tropical Cyclone Report: Hurricane Frances." *National Hurricane Center Tropical Cyclone Report.* http://www.nhc.noaa.gov/2004frances.shtml.

Binstock, Robert H., and Linda K. George. 2011. "Disability, Functioning, and Aging." In *Handbook of Aging and the Social Sciences*, 7th ed. Amsterdam: Elsevier Science & Technology.

Blake, Eric S., Todd B. Kimberlain, Robert J. Berg, John P. Cangialosi, and John L. Beven II. 2013. "Tropical Cyclone Report: Hurricane Sandy." *National Hurricane Center Tropical Cyclone Report.* http://www.nhc.noaa.gov/data/tcr/AL182012_Sandy.pdf.

Blanchard, Gary, and David M. Dosa. 2009. "A Comparison of the Nursing Home Evacuation Experience between Hurricanes Katrina (2005) and Gustav (2008)." *Journal of the American Medical Directors Association* 10 (9): 639–43. doi:10.1016/j.jamda.2009.06.010.

Bland, Thyrie. 2017a. "Hurricane Irma Update: Residents Turned Away from Dunbar High; Shelter Closed." *USA Today*, September 12. https://www.usatoday.com/story/news/2017/09/12/hurricane-irma-dunbar-high-school-opened-shelter/657436001/.

———. 2017b. "Hurricane Irma Update: Lee County Schools Won't Open until Sept. 25." *News Press2*, September 14. http://www.news-press.com/story/news/education/2017/09/14/hurricane-irma-update-lee-county-schools-wont-open-until-sept-25/665896001/.

Bludau, Jurgen. 2010. *Aging But Never Old: The Realities, Myths, and Misrepresentations of the Anti-Aging Movement.* Santa Barbara, CA: Praeger Series on Contemporary Health and Living.

Blumenthal, Herman T. 2003. "The Aging–Disease Dichotomy: True or False?" *Journal of Gerontology A: Biological Sciences and Medical Sciences* 58 (2): M138–45. http://www.ncbi.nlm.nih.gov/pubmed/12586851.

Blustein, Paul, and Craig Timberg. 2005. "High Oil Prices Met with Anger Worldwide." *Washington Post*, October 3. http://www.washingtonpost.com/wp-dyn/content/article/2005/10/02/AR2005100201315.html.

Bolstad, Erika. 2017. "High Ground Is Becoming Hot Property as Sea Level Rises." *Scientific American*, May. https://www.scientificamerican.com/article/high-ground-is-becoming-hot-property-as-sea-level-rises/.

Bonilla, Yarimar. 2018. "How Puerto Ricans Fit into an Increasingly Anti-Immigrant U.S." *Washington Post*, January 19. https://www.washingtonpost.com/news/posteverything/wp/2018/01/19/how-the-u-s-will-replace-immigrant-workers-with-puerto-ricans/?utm_term=.c66659966c24.

"Borehole." 2017. NOAA. Accessed August 18. https://www.ncdc.noaa.gov/data-access/paleoclimatology-data/datasets/borehole.

Borns, Patricia. 2017. "City of Fort Myers Dumped Toxic Sludge in Dunbar." *News Press*, June 26. http://www.news-press.com/story/news/2017/06/12/city-fort-myers-dumped-toxic-sludge-dunbar/369451001/.

Bower, Bruce. 2017. "Ancient Boy's DNA Pushes Back Date of Earliest Humans." *Science News*, September 28. https://www.sciencenews.org/article/ancient-boys-dna-pushes-back-date-earliest-humans.

Brown, Dwayne, Michael Cabbage, and Leslie McCarthy. 2016. "NASA, NOAA Analyses Reveal Record-Shattering Global Warm Temperatures in 2015." https://www.nasa.gov/press-release/nasa-noaa-analyses-reveal-record-shattering-global-warm-temperatures-in-2015.

Brown, Lisa M. 2008. "Issues in Mental Health Care for Older Adults After Disasters." *Generations* 4 (Winter 2007–2008): 21–26.

Brown, Lisa M., Janelle J. Christensen, Anna Ialynytchev, Kali S. Thomas, Kathryn A. Frahm, and Kathryn Hyer. 2015. "Experiences of Assisted Living Facility Staff in Evacuating and Sheltering Residents During Hurricanes." *Current Psychology* 34 (2). doi:10.1007/s1214401593617.

Brown, Lisa M., David M. Dosa, Kali S. Thomas, Kathryn Hyer, Zhanlian Feng, and Vincent Mor. 2012. "The Effects of Evacuation on Nursing Home Residents with Dementia." *American Journal of Alzheimer's Disease and Other Dementias* 27 (6): 406–12. doi:10.1177/1533317512454709.

Brown, Lisa M., Kathryn Hyer, and Lumarie Polivka-West. 2007. "A Comparative Study of Laws, Rules, Codes and Other Influences on Nursing Homes' Disaster Preparedness in the Gulf Coast States." *Behavioral Sciences and the Law* 25 (5): 655–75. doi:10.1002/bsl.

Brulle, Robert J. 2013. "Institutionalizing Delay: Foundation Funding and the Creation of U.S. Climate Change Counter-Movement Organizations." *Climatic Change* 122 (4): 681–94. doi:10.1007/s10584-013-1018-7.

Brumfield, Ben, and Brian Todd. 2014. "The Weather Is Cuckoo This Winter, but There's Method to the Madness." CNN. http://www.cnn.com/2014/02/15/us/weather-weird-pattern/.

Brunkard, Joan, Gonza Namulanda, and Raoult Ratard. 2008. "Research Hurricane Katrina Deaths, Louisiana, 2005." *Disaster Medicine and Public Health Preparedness* 2 (4): 1–9.

Buckley, Cara. 2013. "Twice as Many Structures in FEMA Maps." *New York Times*, January 29. http://www.nytimes.com/2013/01/29/nyregion/homes-in-flood-zone-doubles-in-new-fema-map.html.

Buehler, Ralph, and John Pucher. 2017. "Trends in Walking and Cycling Safety: Recent Evidence from High-Income Countries, with a Focus on the United States and Germany." *American Journal of Public Health* 107 (2): 281–87. doi:10.2105/AJPH.2016.303546.

Bulled, Nicola, and Merrill Singer. 2011. "Syringe-Mediated Syndemics." *AIDS and Behavior* 15 (7): 1539–45. doi:10.1007/s10461-009-9631-1.

Bump, Philip. 2017. "The 'Very Big Ocean' between Here and Puerto Rico Is Not a Perfect Excuse for a Lack of Aid." *Washington Post*, September 26. https://www.washingtonpost.com/news/politics/wp/2017/09/26/the-very-big-ocean-between-here-and-puerto-rico-is-not-a-perfect-excuse-for-a-lack-of-aid/?utm_term=.6bc92f3d0ecc.

Busse, Meghan R., Christopher R. Knittel, and Florian Zettelmeyer. 2012. "Who Is Exposed to Gas Prices? How Gasoline Prices Affect Automobile Manufacturers and Dealerships." NBER Working Paper no. w18610. Cambridge, MA. http://ssrn.com/abstract=2189728.

Button, Gregory V. 2010. *Disaster Culture: Knowledge and Uncertainty in the Wake of Human and Environmental Catastrophe*. Walnut Creek, CA: Left Coast Press.

Cai, Wenju, Guojian Wang, Agus Santoso, Michael J. McPhaden, Lixin Wu, Fei-Fei Jin, Axel Timmermann, et al. 2015. "Increased Frequency of Extreme La Niña Events under Greenhouse Warming." *Nature Climate Change* 5 (2): 132–37. doi:10.1038/nclimate2492.

Callahan, Christopher M., Greg Arling, Wanzhu Tu, Marc B. Rosenman, Steven R. Counsell, Timothy E. Stump, and Hugh C. Hendrie. 2012. "Transitions in Care for Older Adults with and without Dementia." *Journal of the American Geriatrics Society* 60 (5): 813–20. doi:10.1111/j.1532-5415.2012.03905.x.

Campbell, Joseph, with Bill Moyers. 1988. *The Power of Myth*. Based on the PBS series. New York: Doubleday.

Carabello, Ecleen, and Ellie Shechet. 2017. "Nursing Home Owner in Caguas, Puerto Rico: 'There Is No Help.'" *Jezebel*, September. https://jezebel.com/nursing-home-owner-in-caguas-puerto-rico-there-is-no-1818750918.

"Cardiovascular Diseases (CVDs)." 2017. http://www.who.int/mediacentre/factsheets/fs317/en/.

Cardona, Omar Dario, and Marten Van Aast. 2012. "Determinants of Risk: Exposure and Vulnerability." In *Managing the Risks of Extreme Events and Disasters to Advance Climate Change Adaptation*, 65–108. Cambridge: Cambridge University Press.

"Caring for Vulnerable Elders During a Disaster: National Findings of the 2007 Nursing Home Hurricane Summit." 2007. Florida Health Care Assocation.

Carmichael, Wayne W., and Gregory L. Boyer. 2016. "Health Impacts from Cyanobacteria Harmful Algae Blooms: Implications for the North American Great Lakes." *Harmful Algae* 54: 194–212. doi:10.1016/j.hal.2016.02.002.

Carnes, Bruce A., David Staats, and Bradley J. Willcox. 2014. "Impact of Climate Change on Elder Health." *Journal of Gerontology Series A: Biological Sciences and Medical Sciences* 69 (9): 1087–91. doi:10.1093/gerona/glt159.

Castro, Arachu, and Merrill Singer. 2004. *Unhealthy Health Policy: A Critical Anthropological Examination*. Walnut Creek, CA: Alta Mira Press.

Cattell, Maria, and Steven Albert. 2009. "Elders, Ancients, Ancestors and the Modern Life Course." In *The Cultural Context of Aging: Worldwide Perspectives*, edited by Jay Sokolovsky, 115–33. Westport, CT: Praeger.

Cauley, Jane A. 2012. "The Demography of Aging." In *Epidemiology of Aging*, edited by Anne B. Newman and Jane A. Cauley. Dordrecht: Springer Netherlands. doi:10.1007/978-94-007-5061-6.

"Census Transportation Planning Products: The Journey to Work." 2011. *Federal Highway Administration*. http://www.fhwa.dot.gov/planning/census_issues/ctpp/data_products/journey_to_work/jtw1.cfm.

Chan, Gabrielle. 2017. "Australia Recommits to Paris Agreement after Trump's Withdrawal." *Guardian*, June 1. https://www.theguardian.com/environment/2017/jun/02/australia-recom

mits-to-paris-agreement-after-trumps-withdrawal.

Chaney, Eric. 2017. "Puerto Rico Recovery a Tale of Two Islands; Supplies Flowing, but Not to Remote Areas." *Weather.com*, September 27. https://weather.com/storms/hurricane/news/hurricane-maria-puerto-rico-us-virgin-islands-caribbean-impacts-0.

Channel NewAsia. 2018. "Taiwan to Ban Plastic Straws, Cups by 2030." February 22. https://www.channelnewsasia.com/news/asiapacific/taiwan-to-ban-plastic-straws-cups-by-2030-9981998.

Chappell, Bill. 2017. "Geert Wilders, 'Dutch Donald Trump,' Takes Second Place in Closely Watched Election." NPR, March 17. http://www.npr.org/sections/thetwo-way/2017/03/16/520376715/geert-wilders-dutch-donald-trump-takes-second-place-in-closely-watched-election.

Châtel, Francesca de. 2014. "The Role of Drought and Climate Change in the Syrian Uprising: Untangling the Triggers of the Revolution." *Middle Eastern Studies* 50 (4): 521–35. doi:10.1080/00263206.2013.850076.

Chrisafis, Angelique. 2017. "Emmanuel Macron Vows Unity after Winning French Presidential Election." *Guardian*, May 8. https://www.theguardian.com/world/2017/may/07/emmanuel-macron-wins-french-presidency-marine-le-pen.

Christensen, Janelle J. 2012. "Hurricane Preparedness of Community-Dwelling Dementia Caregivers in South Florida." University of South Florida. http://scholarcommons.usf.edu/etd/4010/.

Christensen, Janelle J., E. D. Richey, and Heide Castaneda. 2013. "Seeking Safety: Predictors of Hurricane Evacuation of Community-Dwelling Families Affected by Alzheimer's Disease or a Related Disorder in South Florida." *American Journal of Alzheimer's Disease and Other Dementias* 28 (7): 682–92. doi:10.1177/1533317513500837.

Christensen, Janelle J., Lisa M. Brown, and Kathryn Hyer. 2012. "A Haven of Last Resort: The Consequences of Evacuating Florida Nursing Home Residents to Nonclinical Buildings." *Geriatric Nursing* 33 (5): 375–83. doi:10.1016/j.gerinurse.2012.03.014.

Christian, Michael D., Cindy Hamielec, Neil M. Lazar, Randy S. Wax, Lauren Griffith, Margaret S. Herridge, David Lee, and Deborah J. Cook. 2009. "A Retrospective Cohort Pilot Study to Evaluate a Triage Tool for Use in a Pandemic." *Critical Care* 13 (5): R170. doi:10.1186/cc8146.

Clynes, Tom. 2012. "The Battle over Climate Science." *Popular Science*, June. http://www.popsci.com/science/article/2012-06/battle-over-climate-change.

Cobb, James A. 2013. *Flood of Lies: The St. Rita's Nursing Home Tragedy*. Gretna, LA: Pelican Publishing Company.

Cohen, Lawrence. 1998. *No Aging in India: Alzheimer's, the Bad Family, and Other Modern Things*. Berkeley: University of California Press.

Cole, Steve, and Leslie McCarthy. 2014. "Long-term Global Warming Trend Sustained in 2013." NASA. https://climate.nasa.gov/news/1029/long-term-global-warming-trend-sustained-in-2013/.

———. 2015. "NASA, NOAA Find 2014 Warmest Year in Modern Record." NASA. https://www.nasa.gov/press/2015/january/nasa-determines-2014-warmest-year-in-modern-record.

Coleman, C. Norman, David M. Weinstock, Rocco Casagrande, John L. Hick, Judith L. Bader, Florence Chang, Jeffrey B. Nemhauser, and Ann R. Knebel. 2011. "Triage and Treatment Tools for Use in a Scarce Resources-Crisis Standards of Care Setting after a Nuclear Detonation." *Disaster Medicine and Public Health Preparedness* 5 (S1): S111–21. doi:10.1001/dmp.2011.22.

Colvin, Jill. 2012. "FEMA Redrawing City's Flood Zone After Superstorm Sandy." DNAInfo, December 6. https://www.dnainfo.com/new-york/20121206/new-york-city/fema-redrawing-citys-flood-zone-after-superstorm-sandy.

Connolly, Kate. 2017. "After the US, Far Right Says 2017 Will Be the Year Europe Wakes Up." *Guardian*, January 21. https://www.theguardian.com/world/2017/jan/21/koblenz-far-right-european-political-leaders-meeting-brexit-donald-trump.

"Constitution of Disabled People's International." 1993. http://www.disabledpeoples international.org/Constitution.

Conway, Erik. 2008. "What's in a Name? Global Warming vs. Climate Change." National Aeronautics and Space Administration. http://www.nasa.gov/topics/earth/features/climate_by_any_other_name.html.

Cooper, Jago. 2012. "Fail to Prepare, Then Prepare to Fail: Rethinking Threat, Vulnerability and Mitigation in the Precolumbian Caribbean." In *Surviving Sudden Environmental Climate Change*, edited by Jago Cooper and Payton Sheets, 91. Boulder: University Press of Colorado.

Cooper, Jago, and Payton Sheets. 2012. *Surviving Sudden Environmental Climate Change*. Boulder: University of Colorado.

Cordain, Loren, Janette Brand Miller, S. Boyd Eaton, Neil Mann, Susanne H. A. Holt, and John D. Speth. 2000. "Plant-Animal Subsistence Ratios and Macronutrient Energy Estimations in Worldwide Hunter-Gatherer Diets." *American Journal of Clinical Nutrition* 71 (3): 682–92.

Cordasco, Kristina M., David P. Eisenman, Deborah C. Glik, Joya F. Golden, and Steven M. Asch. 2007. "'They Blew the Levee': Distrust of Authorities Among Hurricane Katrina Evacuees." *Journal of Health Care for the Poor and Underserved* 18 (2): 277–82. doi:10.1353/hpu.2007.0028.

Corell, Robert W. 2008. "The Potential for Rapid Melting of Ice and Amplification of Sea Level Rise." Introduction to Part 2. In *Sudden and Disruptive Climate Change: Exploring the Real Risks and How We Can Avoid Them*, edited by Michael C. MacCracken, Frances Moore, and John C. Topping Jr., 45–46. New York: Earthscan.

Correia, Sónia C., Renato X. Santos, Cristina Carvalho, Susana Cardoso, Emanuel Candeias, Maria S. Santos, Catarina R. Oliveira, and Paula I. Moreira. 2012. "Insulin Signaling, Glucose Metabolism and Mitochondria: Major Players in Alzheimer's Disease and Diabetes Interrelation." *Brain Research* 1441 (March): 64–78. doi:10.1016/j.brainres.2011.12.063.

Coyle, Maureen. 2015. "Understanding Resistance to Climate Change Resistance." *International Journal of Aging* 80 (1). doi:10.1177/0091415015591111.

Cox, P. A., D. A. Davis, D. C. Mash, J. S. Metcalf, and S. A. Banack. 2016. "Dietary Exposure to an Environmental Toxin Triggers Neurofibrillary Tangles and Amyloid Deposits in the Brain." *Proc. R. Soc. B* 283 (1823), p.20152397.

Crate, Susan. 2009. "Gone the Bull of Winter? Contemplating Climate Change's Cultural Implication's in Northeastern Siberia, Russia." In *Anthropology and Climate Change: From Encounters to Actions*, edited by Susan A. Crate and Mark Nuttall, 139–52. Walnut Creek, CA: Left Coast Press.

Crate, Susan A., and Mark Nuttall. 2009. Introduction to *Anthropology and Climate Change: From Encounters to Actions*, edited by Susan A. Crate and Mark Nuttall, 9–38. Walnut Creek, CA: Left Coast Press.

Cummins, Elanor. 2017. "Hurricane Maria's Actual Death Toll May Be 17 Times Higher Than the Current Official Count. The Government Says 62 People Died. The Data Says More Like 1,052." *Slate*, December 8. http://www.slate.com/articles/health_and_science/medical_examiner/2017/12/the_puerto_rican_government_has_likely_underestimated_hurricane_maria_s.html.

Cutter, Susan L. 2003. "The Vulnerability of Science and the Science of Vulnerability." *Annals of the Association of American Geographers* 93 (1): 1–12. doi:10.1111/1467-8306.93101.

"Dangerous By Design 2016." 2017. Smart Growth America. https://smartgrowthamerica.org/dangerous-by-design/.

Dash, Nicole, and Hugh Gladwin. 2007. "Evacuation Decision Making and Behavioral Responses: Individual and Household." *Natural Hazards Review* 8 (3): 69–77. doi:10.1061/(ASCE)1527-6988(2007)8:3(69).

Davenport, Christian, and Gregory Mount. 2007. "Preliminary Results of the Boyer Survey: An Archaeological Investigation Of Lake Okeechobee." West Palm Beach, Florida. http://www.flarchcouncil.org/reports/BoyerSurveyLakeO.pdf.

Davenport, Coral, and Eric Lipton. 2016. "Trump Picks Scott Pruitt, Climate Change Denialist, to Lead E.P.A." *New York Times*, December 7. https://www.nytimes.com/2016/12/07/us/politics/scott-pruitt-epa-trump.html?_r=0.

Davis, Aaron C., Sandhya Somashekhar, Patricia Sullivan, and Perry Stein. 2017. "Moving Florida's Many Seniors out of Irma's Path Has Unique Risks." *Washington Post*, September 9. https://www.washingtonpost.com/national/the-hidden-death-toll-of-hurricane-evacuations/2017/09/09/530fc358-94d6-11e7-89fa-bb822a46da5b_story.html?utm_term=.14ed57ad5ad7.

"Deadly Winter Weather Paralyzes Japan." 2014. *Deutsche Welle*. http://dw.de/p/1B9xZ.

"Deaths Associated with Hurricane Sandy October–November 2012." 2013. *Morbidity and Mortality Weekly Report (MMWR)* 62 (20): 393–97. http://www.cdc.gov/mmwr/preview/mmwrhtml/mm6220a1.htm.

Della-Marta, P. M., J. Luterbacher, H. Weissenfluh, E. Xoplaki, M. Brunet, and H. Wanner. 2007. "Summer Heat Waves over Western Europe 1880–2003, Their Relationship to Large-Scale Forcings and Predictability." *Climate Dynamics* 29 (2–3): 251–75. doi:10.1007/s00382-007-0233-1.

Dennis, Brady. 2016. "Scientists Are Frantically Copying U.S. Climate Data, Fearing It Might Vanish Under Trump." *Washington Post*. https://www.washingtonpost.com/news/energy-environment/wp/2016/12/13/scientists-are-frantically-copying-u-s-climate-data-fearing-it-might-vanish-under-trump/?utm_term=.99019f50f126.

DiJulio, Bianca, Cailey Muñana, and Mollyann Brodie. 2017. "Puerto Rico after Hurricane Maria: The Public's Knowledge and Views of Its Impact and the Response."https://www.kff.org/other/poll-finding/puerto-rico-after-hurricane-maria-the-publics-knowledge-and-views-of-its-impact-and-the-response/.

Donaghy, Timothy, Jennifer Freeman, Francesca Grifo, Karly Kaufman, Tarek Maassarani, and Lexi Shultz. 2007. "Atmosphere of Pressure: Political Interference in Federal Climate Science," 1–82. Union of Concerned Scientists, February 1.

Donat, Markus G., Andrew L. Lowry, Lisa V. Alexander, Paul A. Gorman, and Nicola Maher. 2016. "More Extreme Precipitation in the World's Dry and Wet Regions." *Nature Climate Change* 6 (5): 508–13. doi:10.1038/nclimate2941.

Donnelly, Jeffrey P., and Jonathan D. Woodruff. 2007. "Intense Hurricane Activity over the Past 5,000 Years Controlled by El Niño and the West African Monsoon." *Nature* 447 (7143): 465–68. doi:10.1038/nature05834.

Dooley, Erin. 2017. "Building Codes on Puerto Rico Unable to Withstand Category 5 Storms: Expert." ABC News, September 20. http://abcnews.go.com/US/building-codes-puerto-rico-unable-withstand-category-storms/story?id=49968096.

Dorsey, David. 2017. "Robert E. Lee and Confederate Statues Generate Reverence, Revulsion in Florida." *News Press*, August 18. http://www.news-press.com/story/news/2017/08/18/robert-e-lee-and-confederate-statues-generate-reverence-revulsion-florida/573163001/.

Dosa, David M., Nancy Grossman, Terrie Wetle, and Vincent Mor. 2007. "To Evacuate or Not to Evacuate: Lessons Learned from Louisiana Nursing Home Administrators Following Hurricanes Katrina and Rita." *Journal of the American Medical Directors Association* 8 (3): 142–49. doi:10.1016/j.jamda.2006.11.004.

Dosa, David M., Kathryn Hyer, Lisa M. Brown, Andrew W. Artenstein, Lumarie Polivka-West, and Vincent Mor. 2008. "The Controversy Inherent in Managing Frail Nursing Home Residents during Complex Hurricane Emergencies." *Journal of the American Medical Directors Association* 9 (8): 599–604. doi:10.1016/j.jamda.2008.05.007.

Douglas, Rachel, Ayberk Kocatepe, Anne E. Barrett, Eren Erman Ozguven, and Clayton Gumber. 2017. "Evacuating People and Their Pets: Older Floridians' Need for and Proximity to Pet-Friendly Shelters." *Journals of Gerontology:* Series B, gbx 119. doi: 10.1093/geronb/gbx119.

Doyle, Alister. 2018. "Earth Sweltered Again in 2017: Hottest Year without an El Nino." Reuters. https://www.reuters.com/article/us-climatechange-weather-un/earth-sweltered-aga in-in-2017-hottest-year-without-an-el-nino-idUSKBN1F724I.

Draper, Patricia. 1975. "!Kung Women: Contrasts in Sexual Egalitarianism in Foraging and Sedentary Contexts." In *Toward an Anthropology of Women*, edited by R. R. Rayna, 77–109. New York: Monthly Review Press.

Dressler, Andrew, and Edward A. Parson. 2010. *The Science and Politics of Global Climate Change: A Guide to the Debate*, 2nd ed. Cambridge, MA: Cambridge University Press.

Dumbaugh, Eric, and Yi Zhang. 2013. "The Relationship between Community Design and Crashes Involving Older Drivers and Pedestrians." *Journal of Planning Education and Research* 33 (1): 83–95. doi:10.1177/0739456X12468771.

Eilperin, Juliet, and Brady Dennis. 2017. "Trump Moves Decisively to Wipe Out Obama's Climate-Change Record." *Washington Post*, March 28. https://www.washingtonpost.com/national/health-science/trump-moves-decisively-to-wipe-out-obamas-climate-change-record/2017/03/27/411043d4-132c-11e7-9e4f-09aa75d3ec57_story.html?utm_term=.3a07 19f4e87e.

Eisenman, David P., Kristina M. Cordasco, Steve Asch, Joya F. Golden, and Deborah Glik. 2007. "Disaster Planning and Risk Communication with Vulnerable Communities: Lessons from Hurricane Katrina." *American Journal of Public Health* 97 (Supplement_1): S109–15. doi:10.2105/AJPH.2005.084335.

Eisenman, David P., Deborah Glik, Richard Maranon, Lupe Gonzales, and Steven Asch. 2009. "Developing a Disaster Preparedness Campaign Targeting Low-Income Latino Immigrants: Focus Group Results for Project PREP." *Journal of Health Care for the Poor and Underserved* 20 (2): 330–45. doi:10.1353/hpu.0.0129.

Elert, Emily, and Michael D. Lemonick. 2012. *Global Weirdness: Severe Storms, Deadly Heat Waves, Relentless Drought, Rising Seas and the Weather of the Future*. New York: Pantheon Books.

Elsasser, S. W., and R. E. Dunlap. 2012. "Leading Voices in the Denier Choir: Conservative Columnists' Dismissal of Global Warming and Denigration of Climate Science." *American Behavioral Scientist* 57 (6): 754–76. doi:10.1177/0002764212469800.

Emanuel, Kerry A. 2005. "Increasing Destructiveness of Tropical Cyclones over the Past 30 Years." *Nature* 436 (7051): 686–88. doi:10.1038/nature03906.

———. 2007. "Environmental Factors Affecting Tropical Cyclone Power Dissipation." *Journal of Climate* 20 (22): 5497–5509. doi:10.1175/2007JCLI1571.1.

———. 2012. *What We Know About Climate Change*, 2nd ed. Cambridge, MA: MIT Press.

Estroff, Sue E. 1993. "Identity, Disability, and Schizophrenia: The Problem of Chronicity. Knowledge, Power and Practice." In *Knowledge, Power and Practice*, edited by Shirley Lindenbaum and Margaret Lock, 247. Berkeley: University of California Press.

Estroff, Sue E., David L. Penn, and Julie R. Toporek. 2004. "From Stigma to Discrimination: An Analysis of Community Efforts to Reduce the Negative Consequences of Having a Psychiatric Disorder and Label." *Schizophrenia Bulletin* 30 (3): 493–509. http://www.ncbi. nlm.nih.gov/pubmed/15631242.

Etters, Lynn, Debbie Goodall, and Barbara E Harrison. 2008. "Caregiver Burden among Dementia Patient Caregivers: A Review of the Literature." *Journal of the American Academy of Nurse Practitioners* 20: 423–28. doi:10.1111/j.1745-7599.2008.00342.x.

"Facts About Florida." n.d. http://www.stateofflorida.com/Portal/DesktopDefault.aspx?tabid= 95.

Fagan, Brian. 2004. *The Long Summer: How Climate Changed Civilization*. New York: Basic Books.

———. 2007. *The Little Ice Age: How Climate Made History 1300–1850*. New York: Basic Books.

———. 2008. *The Great Warming: Climate Change and the Rise and Fall of Civilization*. New York: Bloomsbury.

———. 2013. *The Attacking Ocean: The Past, Present, and Future of Rising Sea Levles*. New York: Bloomsbury.

"A Failure of Initiative: Select Bipartisan Committee to Investigate the Preparation for and Response to Hurricane Katrina." 2006. Washington, DC. http://www.katrina.house.gov/.

Falconer, Ian R., and Andrew R. Humpage. 2005. "Health Risk Assessment of Cyanobacterial (Blue-Green Algal) Toxins in Drinking Water." *International Journal of Environmental Research and Public Health* 2 (1):43–50.

Fearnside, Philip M. 2012. "Brazil's Amazon Forest in Mitigating Global Warming: Unresolved Controversies." *Climate Policy* 12 (1): 70–81. doi:10.1080/14693062.2011.581571.

Feere-Sadurni, Luis, Frances Robles, and Lizette Alvarez. 2017. "'This Is Like in War': A Scramble to Care for Puerto Rico's Sick and Injured." *New York Times*, September 26. https://www.nytimes.com/2017/09/26/us/puerto-rico-hurricane-healthcare-hospitals.html? mcubz=3&_r=0.

Fernandez, Lauren S., Deana Byard, Chien-Chih Lin, Samuel Benson, and Joseph A. Barbera. 2002. "Frail Elderly as Disaster Victims: Emergency Management Strategies." *Prehospital and Disaster Medicine* 17 (2): 67–74. http://www.ncbi.nlm.nih.gov/pubmed/12500729.

Fink, Sheri L. 2009a. "Preparing for a Pandemic, State Health Departments Struggle with Rationing Decisions." *ProPublica*, October 24. http://www.propublica.org/article/ preparing-for-a-pandemic-state-health-departments-struggle-rationing-1024.

———. 2009b. "Rationing Medical Care: Health Officials Struggle with Setting Standards." *ProPublica*, December 21. http://www.propublica.org/article/rationing-medical-care-health- officials-struggle-with-setting-standards-122.

———. 2010. "Worst Case: Rethinking Tertiary Triage Protocols in Pandemics and Other Health Emergencies." *Critical Care* 14 (1): 103. doi:10.1186/cc8216.

———. 2012. "Hypothermia and Carbon Monoxide Poisoning Cases Soar in City after Hurricane." *New York Times*, November 29. http://www.nytimes.com/2012/11/29/nyregion/ hypothermia-and-carbon-monoxide-poisoning-cases-soar-in-new-york-after-hurricane- sandy.html.

———. 2013. *Five Days at Memorial: Life and Death in a Storm-Ravaged Hospital*. New York: Crown.

Fiorenza, Luca, Stefano Benazzi, Jeremy Tausch, Ottmar Kullmer, Timothy G. Bromage, and Friedemann Schrenk. 2011. "Molar Macrowear Reveals Neanderthal Eco-Geographic Dietary Variation." *PLoS ONE* 6 (3).

Fischer, Douglas. 2014. "Climate Risks as Conclusive as Link between Smoking and Lung Cancer." *Scientific American*, March. https://www.scientificamerican.com/article/climate-risks-as-conclusive-as-link-between-smoking-and-lung-cancer/.

Fischer, E. M., and R. Knutti. 2015. "Anthropogenic Contribution to Global Occurrence of Heavy-Precipitation and High-Temperature Extremes." *Nature Climate Change* 5 (6): 560–64. doi:10.1038/nclimate2617.

Fjord, Lakshmi. 2007. "Disasters, Race, and Disability: [Un] Seen Through the Political Lens on Katrina." *Journal of Race and Policy* 3 (1): 46–66.

———. 2010. "Making and Unmaking 'Vulnerable Persons': How Disasters Expose and Sustain Structural Inequalities." *Anthropology News* 51 (7): 13–15.

Fjord, Lakshmi, and Lenore Manderson. 2009. "Anthropological Perspectives on Disasters and Disability: An Introduction." *Human Organization* 68 (1): 64–72.

Flemming, Nicholas, Namik Çağatay, Francesco Latino Chiocci, Nena Galanidou, Hauke Jöns, Gilles Lericolais, and Tine Missiaen. 2014. *Land Beneath the Waves: Submerged Landscapes and Sea Level Change: A Joint Geoscience-Humanities Strategy for European Continental Shelf Prehistoric Research*. Oostende: European Marine Board.

"Florida Population by Age Group." 2016. *Population & Demographics*. http://edr.state.fl.us/Content/population-demographics/data/Pop_Census_Day.pdf.

Foley, Katherine Ellen. 2017. "Those 3% of Scientific Papers That Deny Climate Change? A Review Found Them All Flawed." *Quartz*, October 5. https://qz.com/1069298/the-3-of-scientific-papers-that-deny-climate-change-are-all-flawed/.

Folstein, M., S. Folstein, and P. McHugh. 1975. "Mini Mental State: A Practical Method for Grading the Cognitive State of Patients for the Clinician." *Journal of Psychiatric Research* 12: 189–98.

Ford, Donna Y., Tarek C. Grantham, and Gilman W. Whiting. 2008. "Another Look at the Achievement Gap: Learning from the Experiences of Gifted Black Students." *Urban Education* 43 (2). doi:10.1177/0042085907312344.

Fountain, Henry. 2017. "Irma Will Test Florida's Infrastructure, From Dikes to Sewage Plants." *New York Times*, September 9. https://www.nytimes.com/2017/09/09/us/irma-florida-infrastructure-okeechobee.html.

Fowler, Tara, Julia Jacobo, and Emily Shapiro. 2017. "Florida Nursing Home Called Governor's Personal Cellphone for Help." ABC News, September 17. http://abcnews.go.com/US/florida-nursing-home-called-emergency-cellphone-belonging-governors/story?id=49883415.

Francis, Enjoli. 2017. "'We Can't Let Them Die': Caregiver Pleads for Aid for Sick, Elderly in Hurricane-Ravaged Puerto Rico." ABC News, September 22. http://abcnews.go.com/International/die-caregiver-pleads-aid-sick-elderly-hurricane-ravaged/story?id=50025452.

Francis, Jennifer A., and Stephen J. Vavrus. 2012. "Evidence Linking Arctic Amplification to Extreme Weather in Mid-Latitudes." *Geophysical Research Letters* 39 (6). doi:10.1029/2012GL051000.

Frank, Iris C. 2005. "More on the Emergency Response to the Gulf Coast Devastation by Hurricanes Katrina and Rita: Experiences and Impressions." *Journal of Emergency Nursing* 31 (6): 56–62. doi:10.1016/j.jen.2005.10.008.

Fry, Christine L. 2002. "Age." *Encyclopeida of Aging*. http://www.encyclopedia.com/philosophy-and-religion/bible/bible-general/age.

———. 2007. "The Social Construction of Age and the Experience of Aging in the Late Twentieth Century." In *New Dynamics in Old Age: Individual, Environmental and Societal Perspectives*, edited by Hans-Werner Wahl, Clemens Tesch-Romer, and Andreas Hoff. New York: Baywood.

Frye, Marilyn. 1983. "On Being White: Thinking Toward a Feminist Understanding of Race and Race Supremacy." In *The Politics of Reality: Essays in Feminist Theory*. Berkeley, CA: Crossing Press.

Fulop, T., A. Larbi, J. M. Witkowski, J. McElhaney, M. Loeb, A. Mitnitski, and G. Pawelec. 2010. "Aging, Frailty and Age-Related Diseases." *Biogerontology* 11 (5): 547–63. doi:10.1007/s10522-010-9287-2.

Gamble, Janet, and John Balbus. 2016. "The Impacts of Climate Change on Human Health in the United States: A Scientific Assessment." doi:10.7930/J0Q81B0T.

Gamble, Janet, Bradford J. Hurley, Peter A. Schultz, Wendy S. Jaglom, Nisha Krishnan, and Melinda Harris. 2013. "Climate Change and Older Americans: State of the Science." *Environmental Health Perspectives* 121 (1): 15–22. doi:10.1289/ehp.1205223.

Garcia-Navarro, Lulu. 2017. "Recovering from Hurricanes in Texas, Florida, Puerto Rico." *NPR*, September 24. https://www.npr.org/2017/09/24/553253497/recovering-from-hurricanes-in-texas-florida-puerto-rico.

Geggis, Anne, and Aric Chockey. 2017. "Desperation Spreads among Seniors Week after Hurricane Irma." *Sun Sentinel*, September 17. http://www.sun-sentinel.com/news/weather/hurricane/fl-sb-outage-elderly-20170917-story.html.

Getler, Michael. 2015. "Global Warming, Koch and NOVA." *PBS Ombudsman*. http://www.pbs.org/ombudsman/blogs/ombudsman/2015/12/11/global-warming-koch-and-nova/.

Gibbs, Linda I., and Caswell F. Holloway. 2013. "Hurricane Sandy After Action: Report and Recommendations to Mayor Michael R. Bloomberg." May. http://www.nyc.gov/html/recovery/downloads/pdf/sandy_aar_5.2.13.pdf.

Gibson, Carrie. 2017. "How Colonialism and Racism Explain the Inept US Response to Hurricane Maria." *Vox*, October 7. https://www.vox.com/the-big-idea/2017/10/5/16426082/colonialism-racism-american-response-puerto-rico-maria.

Gibson, Mary Jo, and Michele Hayunga. 2006. "We Can Do Better: Lessons Learned for Protecting Older Persons in Disasters." Washington, DC: AARP. http://assets.aarp.org/rgcenter/il/better.pdf.

Giddens, Anthony. 1990. *The Consequences of Modernity*. Stanford, CA: Stanford University Press.

———. 2013. *The Politics of Climate Change*, 2nd ed. Cambridge: Polity Press.

"Global Climate Report—Annual 2013." 2014. National Centers for Environmental Information & NOAA. https://www.ncdc.noaa.gov/sotc/global/201313.

"Global Warming and Hurricanes: An Overview of Current Research Results." 2013. Geophysical Fluid Dynamics Laboratory/NOAA. http://www.gfdl.noaa.gov/global-warming-and-hurricanes.

———. 2017. Princeton. https://www.gfdl.noaa.gov/global-warming-and-hurricanes/.

Gobler, C. J., O. M. Doherty, T. K. Hattenrath-Lehmann, A. W. Griffith, Y. Kang, R. W. and Litaker. 2017. "Ocean Warming since 1982 Has Expanded the Niche of Toxic Algal Blooms in the North Atlantic and North Pacific Oceans." *Proceedings of the National Academy of Sciences*, p.201619575.

González, Catalina, Ligia Estela Urrego, José Ignacio Martínez, Jaime Polanía, and Yusuke Yokoyama. 2010. "Mangrove Dynamics in the Southwestern Caribbean since the 'Little Ice Age': A History of Human and Natural Disturbances." *The Holocene* 20 (6): 849–61. doi:10.1177/0959683610365941.

Gonzalez, George A. 2010. *Urban Sprawl, Global Warming, and the Empire of Capital.* Albany: State University of New York Press.

Greeley, Andrew. 1993. "Religion and Attitudes toward the Environment." *Journal for the Scientific Study of Religion* 32 (1): 19. doi:10.2307/1386911.

Green, Jennifer. 2016. "Archaeomalacological Data and Paleoenvironmental Reconstruction at the Jupiter Inlet I Site (8PB34A), Southeast Florida." Florida Atlantic University. http://fau. digital.flvc.org/islandora/object/fau%3A33457/datastream/OBJ/view/Archaeomalacologi cal_Data_and_Paleoenvironmental_Reconstruction_at_the_Jupiter_Inlet_I_Site__8PB34a___Southeast_Florida.pdf.

Gubrium, Jaber F. 1986. "The Social Preservation of Mind: The Alzheimer's Disease Experience." *Symbolic Interaction* 9 (1): 37–51.

"Guidance on Planning for Personal Assistance Services in General Population Shelters." 2010. Federal Emergency Management Agency. http://www.fema.gov/pdf/emergency/disaster housing/guidance_plan_ps_gpops.pdf.

Guion, Deirdre T., Debra L. Scammon, and Aberdeen Leila Borders. 2007. "Weathering the Storm: A Social Marketing Perspective on Disaster Preparedness and Response with Lessons from Hurricane Katrina." *Journal of Public Policy & Marketing* 26 (1): 20–32. doi:10.1509/jppm.26.1.20.

Ham, Ken. 1998. "A Young Earth—It's Not the Issue!" *USA AiG Newsletter*, January. http:// hannoveribc.com/clientimages/25727/chronological/extrasjanuary/ayoungearthitsnotthe issue.pdf.

Hansen, James, James Powell, Bob Corelle, Kevin Trenberth, Danny Harvey, Eric Chivian, Henry Pollack, et al. 2015. "An Open Letter to Museums from Members of the Scientific Community." Natural History Museum. http://thenaturalhistorymuseum.org/open-letter-to-museums-from-scientists/.

Harkin, Allana. 2017. "What's Happening to Tangier Island?" *Full Frontal with Samantha Bee.* TBS, November 17. https://www.youtube.com/watch?v=WZoVYl9ltcA.

Hashmi, Mahnaz. 2008. "Dementia: An Anthropological Perspective." *International Journal of Geriatric Psychiatry* 24 (2): 207–12. doi:10.1002/gps.2176.

Haviland, William, Harald Prins, Dana Walrath, and Bunny McBride. 2014. *Anthropology: The Human Challenge*, 15th ed. Boston: Cengage.

"Heatwave: A Major Summer Killer." n.d. Weather.gov. https://www.weather.gov/media/ owlie/heatwave.pdf.

Held, Isaac M., and Brian J. Soden. 2000. "Water Vapor Feedback and Global Warming." *Annual Review of Energy and the Environment* 25 (1): 441–75. doi:10.1146/annu rev.energy.25.1.441.

Hendricks, C. Davis, and Jon Hendricks. 1976. "Concepts of Time and Temporal Construction among the Aged, with Implications for Research." In *Time Roles and Self in Old Age*, edited by Jaber Gubrium. New York: Human Sciences Press.

"Herbert Hoover Dike Major Rehabilitation Evaluation Report." 2000. Washington, DC: Corps of Engineers.

Herskovits, Elizabeth. 1995. "Struggling over Subjectivity: Debates about the 'Self' and Alzheimer's Disease." *Medical Anthropology Quarterly* 9 (2): 146–64. doi:10.1525/ maq.1995.9.2.02a00030.

Hevesi, Dennis. 2008. "Frederick Seitz, Physicist Who Led Skeptics of Global Warming, Dies at 96." *New York Times*, March 6. http://www.nytimes.com/2008/03/06/us/06seitz.html? mcubz=3.

Higuera-Gundy, A. M., M. Brenner, D. A. Hodell, et al. 1999. "A 10,300 14C yr Record of Climate and Vegetation Change from Haiti." *Quaternary Research* 52:159–70.

Hitchock, Robert. 2009. "From Local to Global: Perceptions and Realities of Environmental Change Among Kalahari San." In *Anthropology and Climate Change: From Encounters to Action*, 250–61. Walnut Creek, CA: Left Coast Press.

Hodell, D. A., J. H. Curtis, G. A. Jones, et al. 1991. "Reconstruction of Caribbean Climate Change over the Past 10,500 Years." *Nature* 352: 790–93.

Hodges, David. 2017a. "Do Toxic Sites Pose Risk during Irma?" NBC2, September 6. http://www.nbc-2.com/story/36297206/do-toxic-sites-pose-risk-during-irma.

———. 2017b. "Was Your Safety at Risk in Storm Shelters during Hurricane Irma?" NBC2, November 2. http://www.nbc-2.com/story/36751366/was-your-safety-at-risk-in-storm-shel ters-during-hurricane-irma#vuukle-emote.

Hoffman, Kelly M., Sophie Trawalter, Jordan R. Axt, and M. Norman Oliver. 2016. "Racial Bias in Pain Assessment and Treatment Recommendations, and False Beliefs about Biologi- cal Differences between Blacks and Whites." *Proceedings of the National Academy of Sciences* 113 (16): 4296–4301. doi:10.1073/pnas.1516047113.

Hollander, Gail M. 2008. *Raising Cane in the 'Glades: The Global Sugar Trade and the Transformation of Florida*. Chicago: University of Chicago Press.

Honoré, Russel L. 2018. "Leadership Session." Florida Gulf Coast University, March 23.

Hope, Aimie L. B., and Christopher R. Jones. 2014. "The Impact of Religious Faith on Atti- tudes to Environmental Issues and Carbon Capture and Storage (CCS) Technologies: A Mixed Methods Study." *Technology in Society* 38 (August): 48–59. doi:10.1016/ j.techsoc.2014.02.003.

House of Lords. 2017. "Brexit: Environment and Climate Change." House of Lords, European Union Committee. https://publications.parliament.uk/pa/ld201617/ldselect/ldeucom/109/ 109.pdf.

Howell, Nancy. 2010. "Another Look at the !Kung: A Life History Approach." In *Life Histo- ries of the Dobe !Kung Food, Fatness, and Well-Being over the Life-Span*, 1–18. Berkeley: University of California Press.

Hsu, Shi-Ling. 2011. *The Case for a Carbon Tax: Getting Past Our Hang-Ups to Effective Climate Change*. Washington, DC: Island Press.

Huber, Daniel G., and Jay Gulledge. 2011. "Extreme Weather and Climate Change: Under- standing the Link and Managing the Risk." Center for Climate and Energy Solutions.

Hulac, Benjamin. 2016. "Tobacco and Oil Industries Used Same Researchers to Sway Public." *Scientific American*, June. https://www.scientificamerican.com/article/tobacco-and-oil- industries-used-same-researchers-to-sway-public1/.

Hulm, Mike. 2009. *Why We Disagree about Climate Change*. Cambridge, MA: Cambridge University Press.

Huriash, Lisa. 2017. "Florida Death Toll from Hurricane Irma Keeps Rising." *Sun Sentinel*, November 22. http://www.sun-sentinel.com/news/weather/hurricane/fl-reg-hurricane-irma- deaths-20171120-story.html.

Hutton, David. 2008. "Older People in Emergencies: Considerations for Action and Policy Development." World Health Organization.

Hyer, Kathryn, Lisa M. Brown, Janelle J. Christensen, and Kali S. Thomas. 2009. "Weathering the Storm: Challenges to Nurses Providing Care to Nursing Home Residents during Hurri- canes." *Applied Nursing Research: ANR* 22 (4): e9–14. doi:10.1016/j.apnr.2008.11.001.

Hyer, Kathryn, Lumarie Polivka-West, and Lisa M. Brown. 2008. "Nursing Homes and As- sisted Living Facilities: Planning and Decision Making for Sheltering in Place or Evacua- tion." *Generations* (Fall): 29–34.

Ikels, Charlotte. 2002. "Constructing and Deconstructing the Self: Dementia in China." *Journal Of Cross-Cultural Gerontology* 17 (3): 233–51.

Ingram, Lynn. 2013. "California Megaflood: Lessons from a Forgotten Catastrophe." *Scientific American*, January. https://www.scientificamerican.com/article/atmospheric-rivers-califor nia-megaflood-lessons-from-forgotten-catastrophe/.

Jacka, Jerry. 2009. "Global Averages, Local Extremes: The Subtleties and Complexities of Climate Change in Papua New Guinea." In *Anthropology and Climate Change: From Encounters to Actions*, edited by Susan A. Crate and Mark Nuttall. Walnut Creek, CA: Left Coast Press.

Jacobo, Julia. 2017. "25 Years Later: How Florida Buildings Are Better Able to Withstand Category 5 Storms." ABC News, September 6. http://abcnews.go.com/US/25-years-florida-buildings-withstand-category-storms/story?id=49649317.

Jenkins, Pamela, Shirley Laska, and Gretchen Williamson. 2007. "Connecting Future Evacuation to Current Recovery: Saving the Lives of Older People in the Next Catastrophe." *Generations* 31 (4): 49–52.

Jones, Nicola. 2016. "Scientific Challenges Loom for Canada's Trudeau." *Nature* 538 (27): 436. https://www.nature.com/polopoly_fs/1.20868.1477478352!/menu/main/topColumns/topLeftColumn/pdf/538436a.pdf?origin=ppub.

Jonkman, Sebastiaan N., Bob Maaskant, Ezra Boyd, and Marc Lloyd Levitan. "Loss of Life Caused by the Flooding of New Orleans after Hurricane Katrina: Analysis of the Relationship between Flood Characteristics and Mortality." *Risk Analysis: An Official Publication of the Society for Risk Analysis* 29 (5): 676–98. doi:10.1111/j.1539-6924.2008.01190.x.

Jorgensen, Jillian. 2017. "Puerto Rico Deaths Spike after Maria, Raising Questions over Uncounted Hurricane Deaths." *New York Daily News*, November 10. http://www.nydailynews.com/news/national/deaths-spike-puerto-rico-question-maria-death-toll-article-1.3624592.

Jylhä, Kirsti M., Clara Cantal, Nazar Akrami, and Taciano L. Milfont. 2016. "Denial of Anthropogenic Climate Change: Social Dominance Orientation Helps Explain the Conservative Male Effect in Brazil and Sweden." *Personality and Individual Differences* 98 (August): 184–87. doi:10.1016/j.paid.2016.04.020.

Kailes, June, and A. Enders. 2007. "Moving Beyond 'Special Needs': A Function-Based Framework for Emergency Management and Planning." *Journal of Disability Policy Studies* 17 (4): 230–37. doi:10.1177/10442073070170040601.

Kapur, G. Bobby, and Jeffery P. Smith. 2011. *Emergency Public Health: Preparedness and Response.* Edited by G. Bobby Kapur and Jeffery P. Smith. Sadbury, MA: Jones & Bartlett.

Katz, S., A. B. Ford, R. W. Moskowitz, B. A. Jackson, and M. W. Jaffe. 1963. "Studies of Illness in the Aged. The Index of ADL: A Standardized Measure of Biological and Psychosocial Function." *Journal of the American Medical Association* 185:914–19.

Katz, Sidney, Thomas D. Downs, Helen R. Cash, and Robert C. Grotz. 1970. "Progress in Development of the Index of ADL." *Gerontologist* 10 (1 Part 1): 20–30. doi:10.1093/geront/10.1_Part_1.20.

Kaufman, Sharon R. 1988. "Illness, Biography, and the Interpretation of Self Following a Stroke." *Journal of Aging Studies* 2 (3): 217–27. doi:10.1016/0890-4065(88)90002-3.

———. 2006. "Dementia-Near-Death and 'Life Itself.'" In *Thinking about Dementia: Culture, Loss and the Anthropology of Senility*, edited by Annette Leibing and Lawrence Cohen. New Brunswick, NJ: Rutgers University Press.

Kaye, H. Stephen, Charlene Harrington, and Mitchell P. Laplante. 2010. "Long-Term Care: Who Gets It, Who Provides It, Who Pays, and How Much?" *Health Affairs* 29 (1): 11–21. doi:10.1377/hlthaff.2009.0535.

Kelley, Colin P., Shahrzad Mohtadi, Mark A. Cane, Richard Seager, and Yochanan Kushnir. 2015. "Climate Change in the Fertile Crescent and Implications of the Recent Syrian

Drought." *Proceedings of the National Academy of Sciences* 112 (11): 3241–46. doi:10.1073/pnas.1421533112.

Kim, Baek-Min, Seok-Woo Son, Seung-Ki Min, Jee-Hoon Jeong, Seong-Joong Kim, Xiang-dong Zhang, Taehyoun Shim, and Jin-Ho Yoon. 2014. "Weakening of the Stratospheric Polar Vortex by Arctic Sea-Ice Loss." *Nature Communications* 5. Nature Publishing Group: 5646. doi:10.1038/ncomms5646.

Kishore, Nishant, Domingo Marqués, Ayesha Mahmud, Mathew V. Kiang, Irmary Rodriguez, Arlan Fuller, Peggy Ebner, et al. 2018. "Mortality in Puerto Rico after Hurricane Maria." *New England Journal of Medicine* 379 (2): 162–70. doi:10.1056/NEJMsa1803972.

Kitali, A. E., T. Sando, E. E. Ozguven, and R. Moses. 2017. "Understanding the Factors Associated with Severity of Aging Population–Involved Pedestrian Crashes in Florida." *Advances in Transportation Studies* 42 (3): 85–98.

Klas, Mary Ellen. 2017. "Nursing Home Industry Plans Summit in Wake of Governor's Generator Rule." *Miami Herald*, September 17. http://www.miamiherald.com/news/weather/hurricane/article173885516.html.

Klein, Robert, Richard J. Nicholls, and Frank Thomall. 2003. "The Resilience of Coastal Megacities to Weather-Related Hazards." In *Building Safer Cities: The Future of Disaster Risk*, edited by Alcira Kreimer, Margaret Arnold, and Anne Carlin, 101–20. Washington, DC: World Bank.

Kleinberg, Elliot. 2003. *Black Cloud: The Deadly Hurricane of 1928*. New York: Carroll & Graf.

Kleinman, Arthur. 1980. *Patients and Healers in the Context of Culture: An Exploration of the Borderland Between Anthropology, Medicine, and Psychiatry*. Berkeley: University of California Press.

Klinenberg, Eric. 2013. *Heat Wave: A Social Autopsy of Disaster in Chicago*. Chicago: University of Chicago Press.

Knowlton, Kim, Miriam Rotkin-Ellman, Linda Geballe, Wendy Max, and Gina M Solomon. 2011. "Six Climate Change–Related Events in the United States Accounted for about $14 Billion in Lost Lives and Health Costs." *Health Affairs (Project Hope)* 30 (11): 2167–76. doi:10.1377/hlthaff.2011.0229.

Knutson, Thomas R., John L. McBride, Johnny Chan, Kerry A. Emanuel, Greg Holland, Chris Landsea, Isaac Held, James P. Kossin, A. K. Srivastava, and Masato Sugi. 2010. "Tropical Cyclones and Climate Change." *Nature Geoscience* 3 (3): 157–63. doi:10.1038/ngeo779.

Knutson, Thomas R., Joseph J. Sirutis, Ming Zhao, Robert E. Tuleya, Morris Bender, Gabriel A. Vecchi, Gabriele Villarini, and Daniel Chavas. 2015. "Global Projections of Intense Tropical Cyclone Activity for the Late Twenty-First Century from Dynamical Downscaling of CMIP5/RCP4.5 Scenarios." *Journal of Climate* (September). doi:10.1175/JCLI-D-15-0129.1.

Korten, Tristram. 2015. "Gov. Rick Scott's Ban on Climate Change Term Extended to Other State Agencies." *Miami Herald*, March 11. http://www.miamiherald.com/news/state/florida/article13576691.html.

Kossin, James P., Timothy L. Olander, and Kenneth R. Knapp. 2013. "Trend Analysis with a New Global Record of Tropical Cyclone Intensity." *Journal of Climate* 26 (24): 9960–76. doi:10.1175/JCLI-D-13-00262.1.

Kramer, Alexander, Mobarak Hossain Khan, and Heiko J. Jahn. 2011. "Public Health in Megacities and Urban Areas: A Conceptual Framework." In *Health in Megacities and Urban Areas*, edited by Alexander Kramer, Mobarak Hossain Khan, and Frauke Kraas, 3–20. Dordrecht: Springer. doi:10.1007/978-3-7908-2733-0_1.

Kraus, L., E. Lauer, R. Coleman, and A. Houtenville. 2018. "2017 Disability Statistics Annual Report." Durham: University of New Hampshire, Institute on Disability. https:// disabilitycompendium.org/sites/default/files/user-uploads/AnnualReport_2017_FINAL.pdf.

Kreimer, Alcira, Margaret Arnold, and Anne Carlin, eds. 2003. "Building Safer Cities: The Future of Disaster Risk." Disaster Risk Management series, no. 3. Washington, DC: World Bank, 1–299. http://documents.worldbank.org/curated/en/584631468779951316/Building-safer-cities-the-future-of-disaster-risk.

Kundzewicz, Zbigniew W., Shinjiro Kanae, Sonia Seneviratne, et al. 2014. "Flood Risk and Climate Change: Global and Regional Perspectives." *Hydrological Sciences Journal* 59 (1): 1–28. doi:10.1080/02626667.2013.857411.

Kunreuther, Howard, Erwann Michel-Kerjan, and Nicola Ranger. 2012. "Insuring Future Climate Catastrophes." *Climatic Change* 118 (2): 339–54. doi:10.1007/s10584-012-0625-z.

Kurtz, Lauren. 2016. "Climate Scientists Are under Attack from Frivolous Lawsuits." *Guardian*, July 7. https://www.theguardian.com/environment/climate-consensus-97-per-cent/ 2016/jul/07/climate-scientists-are-under-attack-from-frivolous-lawsuits.

Kusenbach, Margarethe, and Carylanna Taylor. 2012. "Hurricane Evacuation among Mobile Home Residents in Florida: The Complex Role of Social Networks." In *Surviving Disaster: The Role of Social Netowrks*, edited by Robin L. Ersing and Kathleeen A. Kost, 63–83. Chicago: Lyceum Books.

Kusisto, Laura, and Arian Campo-Flores. 2017. "Homes Built to Stricter Standards Fared Better in Storm." *Wall Street Journal*, September 16. https://www.wsj.com/articles/one-early-lesson-from-irma-hurricane-building-codes-work-1505559600.

Lackner, Klaus S., Sarah Brennan, Jürg M. Matter, A.-H. Alissa Park, Allen Wright, and Bob van der Zwaan. 2012. "The Urgency of the Development of CO_2 Capture from Ambient Air." *Proceedings of the National Academy of Sciences* 109 (33): 13156–62. doi:10.1073/ pnas.1108765109.

Landesman, Linda Y. 2005. *Public Health Management of Disasters*. Washington, DC: American Public Health Association.

Larsen, C. S., M. C. Griffin, D. L. Hutchinson, V. E. Noble, L. Norr, R. F. Pastor, C. B. Ruff, et al. 2001. "Frontiers of Contact: Bioarcheology of Spanish Florida." *Journal of World Prehistory*. doi:10.1023/A:1011180303211.

Lawton, M. P., and E. M. Brody. 1969. "Assessment of Older People: Self-Maintaining and Instrumental Activities of Daily Living." *Gerontologist* 9:179–86.

Leatherman, S., K. Zhang, and C. Xiao. 2007. "Lake Okeechobee, Florida: The Next Hurricane Disaster?" *Water Resources Impact* 9:5–7.

Leatherman, Stephen. 2006. "10 Most Vulnerable Areas to Hurricanes." *Hurricane Center*. http://www.hurricanecenter.com/hurricane-information/top-10-most-vulnerable-areas-to-hurricanes/.

Lee, Richard B. 1968. "What Hunters Do for a Living, Or, How to Make Out on Scarce Resources." In *Man the Hunter*, edited by R. B. Lee and I. DeVote, 30–41. Chicago: Aldine.

Leibing, Annette. 2006. "Divided Gazes: Alzheimer's Disease, the Person Within, Life and Death." In *Thinking about Dementia: Culture, Loss and the Anthropology of Senility*, edited by Annette Leibing and Lawrence Cohen. New Brunswick, NJ: Rutgers University Press.

Leiserowitz, Anthony. 2006. "Climate Change Risk Perception and Policy Preferences: The Role of Affect, Imagery, and Values." *Climatic Change* 77 (1–2): 45–72. doi:10.1007/ s10584-006-9059-9.

Light, John. 2017. "The Climate Threat Posed by Right-Wing Populism's Rising Tide." *Bill Moyers and Company*, January 17. http://billmoyers.com/story/climate-threat-posed-right-wing-populisms-rising-tide/.

Lima, Joana Madureira, and Sandro Galea. 2018. "Corporate Practices and Health: A Framework and Mechanisms." *Globalization and Health* 14 (1): 21. doi:10.1186/s12992-018-0336-y.

Lin, Ning, Kerry A. Emanuel, Michael Oppenheimer, and Erik Vanmarcke. 2012. "Physically Based Assessment of Hurricane Surge Threat under Climate Change." *Nature Climate Change* 2 (6): 462–67. doi:10.1038/nclimate1389.

Lindell, Michael K. 2013. "Disaster Studies." *Current Sociology* 61 (5–6): 797–825. doi:10.1177/0011392113484456.

Lindzen, Richard. 2009. "Resisting Climate Hysteria." *Quadrant*, June 26. http://quadrant.org.au/opinion/doomed-planet/2009/07/resisting-climate-hysteria/.

Lock, Margaret. 2013. "Making and Remaking Alzheimer Disease." In *The Alzheimer Conundrum: Entanglements of Dementia and Aging*, 26–50. Princeton, NJ: Princeton University Press.

Lopez, German. 2017. "The Research on Race That Could Explain Trump's Slow Response to Puerto Rico." *Vox*, October 3. https://www.vox.com/identities/2017/10/3/16390230/puerto-rico-trump-racism.

Love, Jennifer. 2010. "Approaching 65: A Survey of Baby Boomers Turning 65 Years Old." Washington, DC: AARP.

Luber, George, and Michael McGeehin. 2008. "Climate Change and Extreme Heat Events." *American Journal of Preventive Medicine* 35 (5): 429–35. doi:10.1016/j.amepre.2008.08.021.

Lupton, Deborah. 1993. "Risk as Moral Danger: The Social and Political Functions of Risk Discourses in Public Health." *International Journal of Health Services* 23 (3): 425–35.

———. 1999. *Risk*. New York: Routledge.

Mallick, Bishawjit, Bayes Ahmed, and Joachim Vogt. 2017. "Living with the Risks of Cyclone Disasters in the South-Western Coastal Region of Bangladesh." *Environments* 4 (1): 13. doi:10.3390/environments4010013.

Malinowski, Bronislaw. 1922. *Argonauts of the Western Pacific: An Account of Native Enterprise and Adventure in the Archipelagoes of Melanesian New Guinea*. New York: Dutton. http://www.bohol.ph/books/Argonauts/Argonauts.html.

———. 1967. *A Diary in the Strictest Sense of the Term*, 2nd ed. London: Athlone Press. https://archive.org/stream/MalinowskiBronislawADiaryInTheStrictSenseOfTheTerm/Malinowski+Bronislaw+-+A+Diary+in+the+Strict+Sense+of+the+Term_djvu.txt.

Mann, Michael E., Stefan Rahmstorf, Kai Kornhuber, Byron A. Steinman, Sonya K. Miller, and Dim Coumou. 2017. "Influence of Anthropogenic Climate Change on Planetary Wave Resonance and Extreme Weather Events." *Scientific Reports* 7 (March), no. 45242. doi:10.1038/srep45242.

Mauritsen, Thorsten, and Robert Pincus. 2017. "Committed Warming Inferred from Observations." *Nature Climate Change*. doi:10.1038/nclimate3357.

Mayhorn, Christopher B. 2005. "Cognitive Aging and the Processing of Hazard Information and Disaster Warnings." *Natural Hazards Review* 6 (November): 165–70.

McCann, David G. C. 2011. "A Review of Hurricane Disaster Planning for the Elderly." *World Medical Health Policy* 3 (1): 5–30. doi:10.2202/1948-4682.1144.

McCausland, Phil, and Elizabeth Chuck. 2017. "Hurricane Harvey Evacuations: Residents Warned to Leave, Stay Away." NBC News, August 25. https://www.nbcnews.com/storyline/hurricane-harvey/hurricane-harvey-evacuations-residents-college-students-warned-stay-away-n795891.

McCright, Aaron M., and Riley E. Dunlap. 2011. "Cool Dudes: The Denial of Climate Change among Conservative White Males in the United States." *Global Environmental Change* 21 (4): 1163–72. doi:10.1016/j.gloenvcha.2011.06.003.

McGraw, Meridith, and Sabina Ghebremedhin. 2017. "Hurricane Harvey: Photo of Texas Nursing Home Residents in Waist-Deep Water Prompts Rescue." ABC News, August 27. http://abcnews.go.com/US/hurricane-harvey-photo-texas-nursing-home-residents-waist/story?id=49452958.

McGuinness, B., S. L. Barrett, D. Craig, J. Lawson, and A. P. Passmore. 2010. "Executive Functioning in Alzheimer's Disease and Vascular Dementia." *International Journal of Geriatric Psychiatry* 25 (6): 562–68. doi:10.1002/gps.2375.

McKinney, Nathan, Chris Houser, and Klaus Meyer-Arendt. 2011. "Direct and Indirect Mortality in Florida during the 2004 Hurricane Season." *International Journal of Biometeorology* 55 (4): 533–46. doi:10.1007/s00484-010-0370-9.

McMahon, Paula, Susannah Bryan, and Erika Pesantes. 2017. "Nursing Home Deaths: Hollywood Police Have Search Warrant, Say First Person Died Tuesday." *Sun Sentinel*, September 14. http://www.sun-sentinel.com/local/broward/fl-reg-nursing-home-deaths-20170914-story.html.

McShane, Rupert, Kathy Gedling, Janet Keene, Christopher Fairburn, Robin Jacoby, and Tony Hope. 1998. "Getting Lost in Dementia: A Longitudinal Study of a Behavioral Symptom." *International Psychogeriatrics* 10 (3): 253–60. doi:10.1017/S1041610298005365.

"Meeting of Heads of State and/or Government, NATO Headquarters, 25 May 2017." 2017. http://www.nato.int/cps/en/natohq/events_143956.htm.

Messner, Frank, and Volker Meyer. 2006. "Flood Damage, Vulnerability and Risk Perception-Challenges for Flood Damage Research." In *Flood Risk Management—Hazards, Vulnerability and Mitigation Measures*, edited by Jochen Schanze, Evzen Zeman, and Jiri Marsalek, 149–67. Dordrecht: Springer.

Mhaoláin, Aine M. Ní, Damien Gallagher, Lisa Crosby, Deirdre Ryan, Loretto Lacey, Robert F. Coen, Davis Coakley, J. Bernard Walsh, Conal Cunningham, and Brian Lawlor. 2012. "Frailty and Quality of Life for People with Alzheimer's Dementia and Mild Cognitive Impairment." *American Journal of Alzheimer's Disease and Other Dementias* 27 (1): 48–54. doi:10.1177/1533317511435661.

Miller, Scott D., Michael L. Goulden, Lucy R. Hutyra, Michael Keller, Scott R. Saleska, Steven C. Wofsy, Adelaine Michela Silva Figueira, Humberto R. da Rocha, and Plinio B. de Camargo. 2011. "Reduced Impact Logging Minimally Alters Tropical Rainforest Carbon and Energy Exchange." *Proceedings of the National Academy of Sciences* 108 (48): 19431–35. doi:www.pnas.org/cgi/doi/10.1073/pnas.1105068108.

Milman, Oliver. 2017. "Climate Scientists Face Harassment, Threats and Fears of 'McCarthyist Attacks.'" *Guardian*, February 22. https://www.theguardian.com/environment/2017/feb/22/climate-change-science-attacks-threats-trump.

Min, Seung-Ki, Xuebin Zhang, Francis W. Zwiers, and Gabriele C. Hegerl. 2011. "Human Contribution to More-Intense Precipitation Extremes." *Nature* 470 (7334): 378–81. doi:10.1038/nature09763.

"The Mississippi Flood and Flood Predictions." 1927. *Science* 65 (1688): xii–xiv. doi:10.1126/science.65.1688.0xii.

Monbiot, George. 2006. "The Denial Industry." *Guardian*, September 19. https://www.theguardian.com/environment/2006/sep/19/ethicalliving.g2.

———. 2009. "The Denial Industry Case Notes." *Guardian*, December 7. https://www.theguardian.com/environment/georgemonbiot/2009/dec/07/george-monbiot-blog-climate-denial-industry.

Moody, Harry R. 2015. "Overcoming Objections by Elders to Action on Climate Change." *International Journal of Aging and Human Development* 80 (1): 64–75. doi:10.1177/0091415015591110.

Mooney, Chris. 2007. *Storm World: Hurricanes, Politics, and the Battle Over Global Warming*. Orlando, FL: Harcourt.

Mooney, Chris, and Lisa Rein. 2017. "Don't Call It 'Climate Change': How the Government Is Rebranding in the Age of Trump." *Washington Post*, May 26. https://www.washingtonpost.com/news/energy-environment/wp/2017/05/26/just-dont-call-it-climate-change-rebranding-government-in-the-age-of-trump/?deferJs=true&outputType=default-article&tid=a_inl&utm_term=.fc5e867bbd86.

Moore, Benjamin J., Kelly M. Mahoney, Ellen M. Sukovich, Robert Cifelli, and Thomas M. Hamill. 2015. "Climatology and Environmental Characteristics of Extreme Precipitation Events in the Southeastern United States." *Monthly Weather Review* 143 (3): 718–41. doi:10.1175/MWR-D-14-00065.1.

Morgan, Curtis. 2013. "A Vulnerable Lake Okeechobee." *Maimi Herald*. http://www.miamiherald.com/2013/09/20/3639411/a-vulnerable-lake-okeechobee.html.

Morrison, Mark, Roderick Duncan, and Kevin Parton. 2015. "Religion Does Matter for Climate Change Attitudes and Behavior." Edited by Kristie L. Ebi. *PLOS ONE* 10 (8): e0134868. doi:10.1371/journal.pone.0134868.

Morrow, Betty Hearn. 1999. "Identifying and Mapping Community Vulnerability." *Disasters* 23 (1): 1–18. http://www.ncbi.nlm.nih.gov/pubmed/10204285.

Moser, Patrick. 2004. "US: 2.5 Million Ordered to Flee Homes as Hurricane Frances Bears Down on Florida." *Agence France-Presse*, September 3. http://reliefweb.int/report/united-states-america/us-25-million-ordered-flee-homes-hurricane-frances-bears-down-florida.

Munoz, S. E., K. Gajewski, and M. C. Peros. 2010. "Synchronous Environmental and Cultural Change in the Prehistory of the Northeastern United States." *Proceedings of the National Academy of Sciences* 107 (51): 22008–13. doi:10.1073/pnas.1005764107.

Muramatsu, Naoko, and Hiroko Akiyama. 2011. "Japan: Super-Aging Society Preparing for the Future." *Gerontologist* 51 (4): 425–32. doi:10.1093/geront/gnr067.

Murphy, Brett, and Joseph Cranney. 2017. "'He Was Crying and Moaning in Agony': Public Health Crisis Looms after Irma." *USA Today*, September 17. https://www.usatoday.com/story/news/nation-now/2017/09/17/he-crying-and-moaning-agony-public-health-crisis-looms-after-irma/675822001/.

Murphy, Robert F. 1987. *The Body Silent*. New York: Holt.

Murray, Timothy, and Denis Gaudet. 2013. "Global Change in Winter Climate and Agricultural Sustainability." In *Plant and Microbe Adaptations to Cold in a Changing World*, edited by Ryozo Imai, Midori Yoshida, and Naoyuki Matsumoto, 1–15. New York: Springer Link.

Mykle, Robert. 2002. *Killer 'Cane: The Dealy Hurricane of 1928*. New York: Cooper Square Press.

Nabipour, Iraj, Katayon Vahdat, Seyed Mojtaba Jafari, Raha Pazoki, and Zahra Sanjdideh. 2006. "The Association of Metabolic Syndrome and Chlamydia Pneumoniae, Helicobacter Pylori, Cytomegalovirus, and Herpes Simplex Virus Type 1: The Persian Gulf Healthy Heart Study." *Cardiovascular Diabetology* 5 (January): 25. doi:10.1186/1475-2840-5-25.

National Public Radio. 2013. "How Could a Drought Spark a Civil War?" September 8. https://www.npr.org/2013/09/08/220438728/how-could-a-drought-spark-a-civil-war.

NBC6. 2017. "South Florida Drying Out after Major Flooding in Miami Beach," August 2. http://www.nbcmiami.com/news/local/Heavy-Showers-Cause-Flooding-in-Miami-Beach-437926953.html.

Nedelman, Michael. 2017. "Patients Trapped in Shelters in Puerto Rico Can't Get to Hospitals." *CNN.com*, September 28. http://www.cnn.com/2017/09/28/health/gupta-puerto-rico-hospitals/index.html.

Nedelman, Michael, Steve Almasy, and Emanuella Grinberg. 2017. "At Least 8 Dead after Irma Leaves Florida Nursing Home with No A/C." *CNN.com*, September 13. https://www.cnn.com/2017/09/13/health/florida-nursing-home-deaths/index.html.

Neilan, Brett A., Leanne A. Pearson, Julia Muenchhoff, Michelle C. Moffitt, and Elke Dittmann. 2013. "Environmental Conditions That Influence Toxin Biosynthesis in Cyanobacteria." *Environmental Microbiology* 15 (5): 1239–53. doi:10.1111/j.1462-2920.2012.02729.x.

Nemec, Frank. 2008. "Limited Groundwater Assessment Report: City of Fort Myers Community Development Homerama." Fort Myers. https://www.scribd.com/document/350867461/2008-Dept-of-Environmental-Protection-groundwater-test-report.

"New Orleans, LA, Week of August 28, 2005." 2005. Weather Underground Weather History. https://www.wunderground.com/history/airport/KMSY/2005/9/2/WeeklyHistory.html?&reqdb.zip=&reqdb.magic=&reqdb.wmo=.

New York Times. 2017. "SW Florida Residents Clear Sodden Homes in Scorching Heat." September 18. https://www.nytimes.com/aponline/2017/09/18/us/ap-us-irma-florida.html.

Nichter, Mark. 2003. "Harm Reduction: A Core Concept for Medical Anthropology." In *Risk, Culture, and Health Inequality: Shifting Perceptions of Danger and Blame*, edited by Barbara Herr Harthorn and Laury Oaks, 13. Westport, CT: Praeger.

Noji, Eric K. 2005. "Public Health Issues in Disasters." *Critical Care Medicine* 33 (Supplement): S29–33. doi:10.1097/01.CCM.0000151064.98207.9C.

Nyberg J. B., B. A. Malmgren, A. Kuijpers et al. 2001. "A centennial-Scale Variability of Tropical North Atlantic Surface Hydrography during the Late Holocene." *Palaeogeo P* 183: 25–41.

"Ocean and Coastal Management in Florida." 2012. National Oceanic and Atmospheric Administration Ocean & Coastal Resource Management. http://coastalmanagement.noaa.gov/mystate/fl.html.

Okie, Susan. 2008. "Dr. Pou and the Hurricane—Implications for Patient Care during Disasters." *New England Journal of Medicine* 358 (1): 1–5. doi:10.1056/NEJMp0707917.

O'Laughlin, Daniel T., and John L Hick. 2008. "Ethical Issues in Resource Triage Introduction Ethical Framework Respect for Autonomy Nonmaleficence Beneficence Justice Ethical Dilemmas Tools for Mass-Care Triage Operational Implementation." *Respiratory Care* 53 (2): 190–97.

Oliver, Michael. 1996. *Understanding Disability: From Theory to Practice*. London: Palgrave Macmillan.

Olivera, Gabriela. 2017. "President Trump's Response to Hurricane Maria in Puerto Rico Confirms Second-Class Citizenship." *American Civil Liberties Union*, October 3. https://www.aclu.org/blog/human-rights/president-trumps-response-hurricane-maria-puerto-rico-confirms-second-class.

O'Neill, S., and Sophie Nicholson-Cole. 2009. "'Fear Won't Do It': Promoting Positive Engagement with Climate Change through Visual and Iconic Representations." *Science Communication* 30 (3): 355–79. doi:10.1177/1075547008329201.

Onís, Catalina M. de. 2018. "Energy Colonialism Powers the Ongoing Unnatural Disaster in Puerto Rico." *Frontiers in Communication* 3 (January). doi:10.3389/fcomm.2018.00002.

Oreskes, Naomi, and Erik M. Conway. 2010a. *Merchants of Doubt*. New York: Bloomsbury Press.

———. 2010b. "The Denial of Global Warming." In *Merchants of Doubt*, 169. New York: Bloomsbury Press. https://ncse.com/files/pub/evolution/Excerpt--merchants.pdf.

Ostroff, Caitlin. 2017. "Voicemails from Nursing Home Where 11 Died Were Deleted by Governor's Office." *Miami Herald*, September 24. http://www.miamiherald.com/news/local/community/broward/article175156471.html.

Otkin, Jason A., William E. Lewis, Allen J. Lenzen, Brian D. McNoldy, and Sharanya J. Majumdar. 2017. "Assessing the Accuracy of the Cloud and Water Vapor Fields in the Hurricane WRF (HWRF) Model Using Satellite Infrared Brightness Temperatures." doi:10.1175/MWR-D-16-0354.1.

"Paris Agreement—Status of Ratification." 2016. *UNFCCC*. http://unfccc.int/paris_agreement/items/9444.php.

Parks, Miles. 2017. "Confederate Statues Were Built to Further a 'White Supremacist Future.'" NPR, August 20. http://www.npr.org/2017/08/20/544266880/confederate-statues-were-built-to-further-a-white-supremacist-future.

Pasch, Richard J., Daniel P. Brown, and Eric S. Blake. 2011. "Tropical Cyclone Report: Hurricane Charley." *National Hurricane Center Tropical Cyclone Report*. http://www.nhc.noaa.gov/pdf/TCR-AL032004_Charley.pdf.

Patin, Etienne, Guillaume Laval, Luis B. Barreiro, Antonio Salas, Ornella Semino, Silvana Santachiara-Benerecetti, Kenneth K. Kidd, et al. 2009. "Inferring the Demographic History of African Farmers and Pygmy Hunter–Gatherers Using a Multilocus Resequencing Data Set." Edited by Anna Di Rienzo. *PLoS Genetics* 5 (4): e1000448. doi:10.1371/journal.pgen.1000448.

Pearce, Annie, and Yong Ahn. 2017. *Sustainable Buildings and Infrastructure: Paths to the Future*, 2nd ed. Abingdon: Routledge.

Peros, Matthew, Braden Gregory, Felipe Matos, Eduard Reinhardt, and Joseph Desloges. 2015. "Late-Holocene Record of Lagoon Evolution, Climate Change, and Hurricane Activity from Southeastern Cuba." *The Holocene* 25 (9): 1483–97. doi:10.1177/0959683615585844.

Petoukhov, Vladimir, and Vladimir A. Semenov. 2010. "A Link between Reduced Barents-Kara Sea Ice and Cold Winter Extremes over Northern Continents." *Journal of Geophysical Research* 115 (D21): D21111. doi:10.1029/2009JD013568.

Phifer, James F. 1990. "Psychological Distress and Somatic Symptoms after Natural Disaster: Differential Vulnerability among Older Adults." *Psychology and Aging* 5 (3): 412–20.

Phifer, James F., Krzysztof Kaniasty, and Fran Norris. 1988. "The Impact of Natural Disaster on the Health of Older Adults: A Multiwave Prospective Study." *Journal of Health and Social Behavior* 29 (1): 65–78.

Pillemer, Karl, Nancy M. Wells, Linda P. Wagenet, Rhoda H. Meador, and Jennifer T. Parise. 2011. "Environmental Sustainability in an Aging Society: A Research Agenda." *Journal of Aging and Health* 23 (3): 433–53. doi:10.1177/0898264310381278.

Polzin, Steven E., Alan E. Pisarski, and Penelope Weinberger. 2013. "Commuting in America 2013." American Association of State Highway and Transportation Officials. http://traveltrends.transportation.org/Documents/B7_Vehicle and Transit Availability_CA07-4_web.pdf.

Pongiglione, Francesca. 2012. "Anthropology and Climate Change: From Encounters to Actions; Political Theory and Global Climate Change Ethics, Policy & Environment." *Ethics, Policy & Environment* 15 (1): 125–29.

Potter, Sean, Michael Cabbage, and Leslie McCarthy. 2017. "NASA, NOAA Data Show 2016 Warmest Year on Record Globally." NASA, January 18. https://www.nasa.gov/press-release/nasa-noaa-data-show-2016-warmest-year-on-record-globally.

Poumadère, Marc, Claire Mays, Sophie Le Mer, and Russell Blong. 2005. "The 2003 Heat Wave in France: Dangerous Climate Change Here and Now." *Risk Analysis: An Official*

Publication of the Society for Risk Analysis 25 (6): 1483–94. doi:10.1111/j.1539-6924.2005.00694.x.

Profita, Cassandra, and Jes Burns. 2017. "Recycling Chaos in U.S. as China Bans 'Foreign Waste.'" National Public Radio, December 9. https://www.npr.org/2017/12/09/568797388/recycling-chaos-in-u-s-as-china-bans-foreign-waste.

Prohaska, Thomas R., Lynda A. Anderson, and Robert H. Binstock, eds. 2012. *Public Health for an Aging Society*. Baltimore: Johns Hopkins University Press.

Radcliffe, Ron. 2011. "Stand Up and Be Counted!" *Alzheimer's Community Care Quarterly Magazine*, December. http://cdn.trustedpartner.com/docs/library/AlzheimersCommunityCare2012/news/ACC_Winter_Qtly-WEB.pdf.

Readfearn, Graham. 2017. "Ten Years Ago, Turnbull Called Out Peter Garrett on Climate. What Went Wrong?" *Guardian*, June 20. https://www.theguardian.com/environment/planet-oz/2017/jun/21/ten-years-ago-turnbull-called-out-peter-garrett-on-climate-what-went-wrong.

Reed, Andra J., Michael E. Mann, Kerry A. Emanuel, and David W. Titley. 2015. "An Analysis of Long-Term Relationships among Count Statistics and Metrics of Synthetic Tropical Cyclones Downscaled from CMIP5 Models." *Journal of Geophysical Research: Atmospheres* 120 (15): 7506–19. doi:10.1002/2015JD023357.

"Region II Coastal Analysis and Mapping." n.d. FEMA. http://www.region2coastal.com/.

Resnick, Brian, and Eliza Barclay. 2017. "What Every American Needs to Know about Puerto Rico's Hurricane Disaster." *Vox*, September 28. https://www.vox.com/science-and-health/2017/9/26/16365994/hurricane-maria-2017-puerto-rico-san-juan-humanitarian-disaster-electricty-fuel-flights-facts.

Revesz, Rachael. 2017. "UK to 'Scale Down' Climate Change and Illegal Wildlife Measures to Bring in Post-Brexit Trade, Secret Documents Reveal." *Independent*, November 9. http://www.independent.co.uk/news/uk/politics/uk-government-to-scale-down-climate-change-and-illegal-wildlife-measure-a7674706.html.

Rice, Doyal. 2016. "Greenland's Ice Melting Faster Than We Thought, Study Finds." *USA Today*, September 22. https://www.usatoday.com/story/weather/2016/09/22/greenlands-ice-melting-faster-than-we-thought-study-finds/90841276/.

Richmond, Ashley. 2017. "Gov. Scott Institutes New Rules Following Irma Deaths." WTXL ABC, September 17. http://www.wtxl.com/news/gov-scott-institutes-new-rules-following-irma-deaths/article_91c22426-9bfa-11e7-a994-dfcc5f337860.html?utm_medium=social&utm_source=twitter&utm_campaign=user-share.

Rignot, E., I. Velicogna, M. R. van den Broeke, A. Monaghan, and J. T. M. Lenaerts. 2011. "Acceleration of the Contribution of the Greenland and Antarctic Ice Sheets to Sea Level Rise." *Geophysical Research Letters* 38 (5): n/a-n/a. doi:10.1029/2011GL046583.

Risher, John F., G. Daniel Todd, Dean Meyer, and Christie L. Zunker. 2010. "The Elderly as a Sensitive Population in Environmental Exposures: Making the Case." *Reviews of Environmental Contamination and Toxicology* 207:95–157. http://search.ebscohost.com/login.aspx?direct=true&db=cmedm&AN=20652665&site=ehost-live.

Robine, J. M., S. L. Cheung, S. Le Roy, H. Van Oyen, and F. R. Herrmann. 2007. "Report on Excess Mortality in Europe during Summer 2003 (EU Community Action Programme for Public Health, Grant Agreement 2005114)." http://ec.europa.eu/health/ph_projects/2005/action1/docs/action1_2005_a2_15_en.pdf.

Robinson, L., D. Hutchings, L. Corner, T. Finch, J. Hughes, K. Brittain, and J. Bond. 2007. "Balancing Rights and Risks: Conflicting Perspectives in the Management of Wandering in Dementia." *Health, Risk & Society* 9 (4): 389–406. doi:10.1080/13698570701612774.

Robles, Frances. 2017. "Puerto Rico Deaths Spike, but Few Are Attributed to Hurricane." *New York Times*, November 8. https://www.nytimes.com/2017/11/08/us/puerto-rico-deaths-fema.html.

Robles, Frances, Keenan Davis, Sheri Fink, and Sarah Almukhtar. 2017. "Official Toll in Puerto Rico: 64. Actual Deaths May Be 1,052." *New York Times*, December 9. https://www.nytimes.com/interactive/2017/12/08/us/puerto-rico-hurricane-maria-death-toll.html.

Robles, Frances, and Luis Ferre-Sadurni. 2017. "Puerto Rico's Agriculture and Farmers Decimated by Maria." *New York Times*, September 24. https://www.nytimes.com/2017/09/24/us/puerto-rico-hurricane-maria-agriculture-.html.

Rodgers, Lucy, David Gritten, James Offer, and Patrick Asare. 2016. "Syria: The Story of the Conflict." BBC News, March 11. http://www.bbc.com/news/world-middle-east-26116868.

Romieu, E., T. Welle, S. Schneiderbauer, M. Pelling, and C. Vinchon. 2010. "Vulnerability Assessment within Climate Change and Natural Hazard Contexts: Revealing Gaps and Synergies through Coastal Applications." *Sustainability Science* 5 (2): 159–70. doi:10.1007/s11625-010-0112-2.

Rose, Lily. 2018. "Taiwan Plans to Ban Plastic Straws, Bags, and Utensils by 2030." *Los Angeles Times*, February 22. http://www.latimes.com/food/sns-dailymeal-1888556-eat-taiwan-bans-plastic-straws-bags-utensils-022218-20180222-story.html.

Rosenberg, Katherine. 2014. "Supreme Court Ruling to Integrate Schools Didn't Affect SWFL until a Decade Later." *Naples News*, May 17. http://archive.naplesnews.com/news/education/supreme-court-ruling-to-integrate-schools-didnt-affect-swfl-until-a-decade-later-ep-505424841-341259901.html/.

Rothman, Marc, and Lisa M. Brown. 2006. "The Vulnerable Geriatric Casualty: Medical Needs of Frail Older Adults During Disasters." *Generations* 31 (4): 16–20.

Rowe, Meredeth A., Sydney S. Vandeveer, Catherine A. Greenblum, Cassandra N. List, Rachael M. Fernandez, Natalie E. Mixson, and Hyo C. Ahn. 2011. "Persons with Dementia Missing in the Community: Is It Wandering or Something Unique?" *BMC Geriatrics* 11 (1). BioMed Central Ltd: 28. doi:10.1186/1471-2318-11-28.

Sandweiss, Daniel, and Daniel Quilter. 2012. "Collation, Correlation, and Causation in the Prehistory of Coastal Peru." In *Surviving Sudden Environmental Climate Change*, edited by Jago Cooper and Payton Sheets, 117. Boulder: University Press of Colorado.

Sarkissian, Arek. 2017. "11th Resident of South Florida Nursing Home Dies." *USA Today*, September 23. https://www.usatoday.com/story/news/nation-now/2017/09/23/11-th-resident-south-florida-nursing-home-dies/695944001/.

Sassaman, Kenneth E., Neill J. Wallis, Paulette S. McFadden, Ginessa J. Mahar, Jessica A. Jenkins, Mark C. Donop, Micah P. Monés, et al. 2017. "Keeping Pace with Rising Sea: The First 6 Years of the Lower Suwannee Archaeological Survey, Gulf Coastal Florida." *Journal of Island and Coastal Archaeology* 12 (2): 173–99. doi:10.1080/1556489 4.2016.1163758.

Satariano, William A., Jack M. Guralnik, Richard J. Jackson, Richard A. Marottoli, Elizabeth A. Phelan, and Thomas R. Prohaska. 2012. "Mobility and Aging: New Directions for Public Health Action." *American Journal of Public Health* 102 (8): 1508–15. doi:10.2105/AJPH.2011.300631.

Sauerborn, Rainer, and Kristie L. Ebi. 2012. "Climate Change and Natural Disasters: Integrating Science and Practice to Protect Health." *Global Health Action* 5 (December). doi:10.3402/gha.v5i0.19295.

Schinka, John A., Lisa M. Brown, and Zoe Proctor-Weber. 2009. "Measuring Change in Everyday Cognition: Development and Initial Validation of the Cognitive Change Checklist (3CL)." *American Journal of Geriatric Psychiatry* 17 (6): 516–25.

Schlebusch, Carina M., Helena Malmström, Torsten Günther, Per Sjödin, Alexandra Coutinho, Hanna Edlund, Arielle R. Munters, et al. 2017. "Ancient Genomes from Southern Africa Pushes Modern Human Divergence beyond 260,000 Years Ago." *bioRxiv*. doi:10.1101/145409.

Schleifstein, Mark. 2009. "Study of Hurricane Katrina's Dead Shows Most Were Old, Lived Near Levee Breaches." *Times-Picayune*, August 27. http://www.nola.com/hurricane/index.ssf/2009/08/answers_are_scarce_in_study_of.html.

Schneider, Alexandra, Susanne Breitner, Irene Bruske, Kathrin Wolf, Regina Ruckerl, and Annette Peters. 2011. "Health Effects of Air Pollution and Air Temperature." In *Health in Megacities and Urban Areas*, edited by Alexander Kramer, Mobarak Hossain Khan, and Frauke Kraas, 119–33. Dordrecht: Springer.

Scott, Shirley V. 2008. "Securitizing Climate Change: International Legal Implications and Obstacles." *Cambridge Review of International Affairs* 21 (4): 603–19. doi:10.1080/09557570802452946.

Schultz, P. Wesley, Lynnette Zelezny, and Nancy J. Dalrymple. 2000. "A Multinational Perspective on the Relation between Judeo-Christian Religious Beliefs and Attitudes of Environmental Concern." *Environment and Behavior* 32 (4): 576–91.

Science News. 2017. "Florida Flood Risk Study Identifies Priorities for Property Buyouts." August. https://www.sciencedaily.com/releases/2017/08/170817092825.htm.

Semenza, Jan C., Jonathan E. Suk, Virginia Estevez, Kristie L. Ebi, and Elisabet Lindgren. 2012. "Mapping Climate Change Vulnerabilities to Infectious Diseases in Europe." *Environmental Health Perspectives* 120 (3): 385–92.

Shah, Kaushik, Shanal Desilva, and Thomas Abbruscato. 2012. "The Role of Glucose Transporters in Brain Disease: Diabetes and Alzheimer's Disease." *International Journal of Molecular Sciences* 13 (10): 12629–55. doi:10.3390/ijms131012629.

Shapiro, Emily, and Julia Jacobo. 2017. "Florida Nursing Home Patients Had Body Temperatures of up to 106 Degrees, Officials Say." ABC News, September 14. http://abcnews.go.com/US/florida-nursing-home-victim-told-friend-breathe-day/story?id=49844951.

Shear, Michael. 2017. "Trump Will Withdraw U.S. from Paris Climate Agreement." *New York Times*, June 1. https://www.nytimes.com/2017/06/01/climate/trump-paris-climate-agreement.html.

"Shell Point Pricing." 2017. Shell Point. http://www.shellpoint.org/pricing/.

Shultz, James M., Jill Russell, and Zelde Espinel. 2005. "Epidemiology of Tropical Cyclones: The Dynamics of Disaster, Disease, and Development." *Epidemiologic Reviews* 27 (1): 21–35. doi:10.1093/epirev/mxi011.

Singer, Merrill. 2008. "The Perfect Epidemiological Storm: Food Insecurity, HIV/AIDS and Poverty in Southern Africa." *Anthropology News* 49(7):12, 15.

———. 2009. *Introduction to Syndemics: A Critical Systems Approach to Public and Community Health*. San Francisco: Jossey-Bass.

———. 2010. "Ecosyndemics: Global Warming and the Coming Plagues of the Twenty-First Century." In *Plagues and Epidemics: Infected Spaces Past and Present*, edited by D. Ann Herring and Alan C. Swedlund, 21–38. Oxford: Berg.

———. 2013. "Respiratory Health and Ecosyndemics in a Time of Global Warming." *Health Sociology Review* 22 (1): 98–111.

Singer, Merrill, and Hans A. Baer. 2009. "Introduction: Hidden Harm: The Complex World of Killer Commodities." In *Killer Commodities: Public Health and the Corporate Production of Harm*, edited by Merrill Singer and Hans Baer, 1–34. Plymouth, UK: AltaMira Press.

———. 2016. "Applied Medical Anthropology and the Adverse Health Effects of Climate Change." In *Understanding and Applying Medical Anthropology: Biosocial and Cultural*

Approaches, edited by Peter J. Brown and Svea Closser, 3rd ed., 106–16. New York: Taylor and Francis.

Singer, Merrill, and Scott Clair. 2003. "Syndemics and Public Health: Reconceptualizing Disease in Bio-Social Context." *Medical Anthropology Quarterly* 17 (4): 423–41. http://www.ncbi.nlm.nih.gov/pubmed/14716917.

Singer, Merrill, Pamela I. Erickson, Louise Badiane, Rosemary Diaz, Dugeidy Ortiz, Traci Abraham, and Anna Marie Nicolaysen. 2006. "Syndemics, Sex and the City: Understanding Sexually Transmitted Diseases in Social and Cultural Context." *Social Science & Medicine (1982)* 63 (8): 2010–21. doi:10.1016/j.socscimed.2006.05.012.

Smith, Ashley A. 2014. "Lee Lagged on Integration." *News Press*, May 17. http://www.news-press.com/story/news/education/2014/05/16/lee-lagged-integration/9197985/.

Smith, N., and A. Leiserowitz. 2013. "American Evangelicals and Global Warming." *Global Environmental Change* 23 (5): 1009–17. doi:10.1016/j.gloenvcha.2013.04.001.

Snell, Bradford. 1974. "American Ground Transport." In *Crisis in American Institutions*, edited by Jerome Skolnick and Elliott Currie, 276–89. http://www.math.uci.edu/~brusso/Snell1974_645.rtf.

Solimeo, Samantha. 2009. *With Shaking Hands: Aging with Parkinson's Disease in America's Heartland*. New Brunswick, NJ: Rutgers University Press.

Solomon, David. 1999. "The Role of the Aging Process in Aging-Dependent Diseases." In *Handbook of Theories of Aging*, edited by Vern L. Bengtson and K. Warner Schaie, 133–50. New York: Springer.

Solomon, Paul R., Aliina Hirschoff, Bridget Kelly, Mahri Relin, Michael Brush, Richard D. Deveaux, and William W. Pendlebury. 1998. "A 7-Minute Neurocognitive Screening Battery Highly Sensitive to Alzheimer's Disease." *Archeological Neurology* 55:349–55.

Solomon, S., D. Qin, M. Manning, Z. Chen, M. Marquis, K. B. Averyt, M. Tignor, and H. L. Miller, eds. 2007. "Observations: Surface Atmospheric Climate Change." In *Contribution of Working Group I to the Fourth Assessment Report of the Intergovernmental Panel on Climate Change*. Cambridge: Cambridge University Press. http://www.ipcc.ch/publications_and_data/publications_ipcc_fourth_assessment_report_wg1_report_the_physical_science_basis.htm.

Sorensen, John H. 2000. "Hazard Warning Systems: Review of 20 Years of Progress." *Natural Hazards Review* 1 (2): 119–25.

Sorensen, John H., and Barbara Vogt Sorensen. 2007. "Community Processes: Warning and Evacuation." In *Handbook of Disaster Research*, edited by Havidán Rodríguez, Enrico L. Quarantelli, and Russell R. Dynes, 183–99. New York: Springer.

"Special Needs Shelter Program." 2017. Florida Department of Health. Accessed January 2. http://www.floridahealth.gov/programs-and-services/emergency-preparedness-and-response/healthcare-system-preparedness/spns-healthcare/index.html.

"Speleothem and Caves." 2017. NOAA. Accessed August 18. https://www.ncdc.noaa.gov/data-access/paleoclimatology-data/datasets/speleothem.

Spencer, Terry, Jennifer Kay, and Tim Reynolds. 2017. "'Red Flag' Calls Signaled Post-Irma Deaths at Nursing Home." *Miami Herald*, September 16. http://www.miamiherald.com/news/article173687096.html.

Speth, John D. 1990. "Seasonality, Resource Stress, and Food Sharing in So-Called 'Egalitarian' Foraging Societies." *Journal of Anthropological Archaeology* 9 (2): 148–88. doi:10.1016/0278-4165(90)90002-U.

Sprung, Charles L., Marion Danis, Gaetano Iapichino, Antonio Artigas, Jozef Kesecioglu, Rui Moreno, Anne Lippert, et al. 2013. "Triage of Intensive Care Patients: Identifying Agreement and Controversy." *Intensive Care Medicine* 39 (11): 1916–24. doi:10.1007/s00134-013-3033-6.

Stanton, Elizabeth A, and Frank Ackerman. 2007. "Florida and Climate Change: The Costs of Inaction." Global Development and Environment Institute, Tufts University.

Stapleton, Christine. 2017. "With Lake Okeechobee on Way to 10-Year High, Corps Releases Water East." *Palm Beach Post*, September 14. http://www.palmbeachpost.com/news/with-lake-okeechobee-way-year-high-corps-releases-water-east/CjWYAQzXzYHMsP3qnu OAZN/.

Stein, Julie K. 1986. "Coring Archaeological Sites." *American Antiquity* 51 (3): 505–27. doi:10.2307/281749.

Stern, Roger J. 2010. "United States Cost of Military Force Projection in the Persian Gulf, 1976–2007." *Energy Policy* 38 (6): 2816–25. doi:10.1016/j.enpol.2010.01.013.

Stewart, John. 2014. "War on Carbon: *The Daily Show with John Stewart*." Comedy Central. http://www.thedailyshow.com/watch/mon-january-6-2014/war-on-carbon.

Stewart, Stacy R. 2005. "Tropical Cyclone Report: Hurrican Ivan." *National Hurricane Center Tropical Cyclone Report*. http://www.nhc.noaa.gov/2004ivan.shtml.

Stommel, E. W., N. C. Field, T. A., and Caller. 2013. "Aerosolization of Cyanobacteria as a Risk Factor for Amyotrophic Lateral Sclerosis." *Medical Hypotheses* 80 (2):142–45.

Stone, Brian. 2012. *The City and the Coming Climate: Climate Change in the Places We Live*. Cambridge, MA: Cambridge University Press.

Stopford, Cheryl L., Jennifer C. Thompson, David Neary, Anna M. T. Richardson, and Julie S. Snowden. 2012. "Working Memory, Attention, and Executive Function in Alzheimer's Disease and Frontotemporal Dementia." *Cortex: A Journal Devoted to the Study of the Nervous System and Behavior* 48 (4): 429–46. doi:10.1016/j.cortex.2010.12.002.

Stott, Peter A., D. A. Stone, and M. R. Allen. 2004. "Human Contribution to the European Heatwave of 2003." *Nature* 432 (7017): 610–14. doi:10.1038/nature03089.

Subaiya, Saleena, Cyrus Moussavi, Anthony Velasquez, and Joshua Stillman. 2014. "A Rapid Needs Assessment of the Rockaway Peninsula in New York City after Hurricane Sandy and the Relationship of Socioeconomic Status to Recovery." *American Journal of Public Health* 104 (4): 632–38.

Supran, Geoffrey, and Naomi Oreskes. 2017. "Assessing ExxonMobil's Climage Change Communications." Environmental Research Letters 12 (8): 1–18. doi:10.1088/1748-9326/aa815f.

Sutter, John. 2017. "Researchers Raise New Questions about the Hurricane Death Toll in Puerto Rico." CNN, November 29. https://www.cnn.com/2017/11/29/health/demographers-puerto-rico-death-toll-estimatLIne-invs/index.html.

Swenson, Kyle. 2017. "Florida Governor's Office Deleted Critical Messages Related to Post-Hurricane Nursing Home Deaths." *Washington Post*, September 25. https://www.washingtonpost.com/news/morning-mix/wp/2017/09/25/florida-governor-deleted-critical-emails-related-to-post-hurricane-nursing-home-deaths/?utm_term=.c09e7b45f958.

"Syria Emergency." 2018. United Nations Refugee Agency UNHCR. http://www.unhcr.org/en-us/syria-emergency.html.

Tankersley, Jim, and Chris Mooney. 2016. "What Charles Koch Really Thinks about Climate Change." *Washington Post*, June 6. https://www.washingtonpost.com/news/energy-environment/wp/2016/06/06/what-charles-koch-really-thinks-about-climate-change/?utm_term=.4c5c9c791f17.

Taylor, Richard. 2007. *Alzheimer's from the Inside Out*. Baltimore: Health Professions Press.

Teunisse, S., and M. M. Derix. 1997. "The Interview for Deterioration in Daily Living Activities in Dementia: Agreement between Primary and Secondary Caregivers." *International*

Psychogeriatrics / IPA 9 Suppl 1 (January): 155–62. http://www.ncbi.nlm.nih.gov/pubmed/9447438.

Thomas, Kali S., Kathryn Hyer, Lisa M. Brown, LuMarie Polivka-West, and Laurence G. Branch. 2010. "Florida's Model of Nursing Home Medicaid Reimbursement for Disaster-Related Expenses." *Gerontologist* 50 (2): 263–70. doi:10.1093/geront/gnp132.

Thomas, S. B., and S. C. Quinn. 1991. "The Tuskegee Syphilis Study, 1932 to 1972: Implications for HIV Education and AIDS Risk Education Programs in the Black Community." *American Journal of Public Health* 81 (11): 1498–504. doi:10.2105/Ajph.81.11.1498.

Thompson, Victor D., and Thomas J. Pluckhahn. 2010. "History, Complex Hunter-Gatherers, and the Mounds and Monuments of Crystal River, Florida, USA: A Geophysical Perspective." *Journal of Island and Coastal Archaeology* 5 (1): 33–51. doi:10.1080/1556489090 3249811.

Tollefson, Jeff. 2017. "Trump's Pick for Secretary of State Backs Paris Climate Accord." *Scientific American*, January 12. https://www.scientificamerican.com/article/trumps-pick-for-secretary-of-state-backs-paris-climate-accord/%0A%0A.

Trenberth, Kevin. 2007. "Warmer Oceans, Stronger Hurricanes: Evidence Is Mounting That Global Warming Enhances a Cyclone's Damaging Winds and Flooding Rains." *Scientific American* 297 (1): 44–51.

———. 2011. "Changes in Precipitation with Climate Change." *Climate Research* 47 (1–2): 123–38. doi:10.3354/cr00953.

———. 2012. "Framing the Way to Relate Climate Extremes to Climate Change." *Climatic Change* 115 (2): 283–90. doi:10.1007/s10584-012-0441-5.

Truscott, Roger J. W., and Xiangjia Zhu. 2010. "Presbyopia and Cataract: A Question of Heat and Time." *Progress in Retinal and Eye Research* 29 (6): 487–99. doi:10.1016/j.preteyeres.2010.05.002.

Tsikoudakis, Mike. 2012. "Hurricane Andrew Prompted Better Building Code Requirements." *Business Insurance*, August 19. https://www.businessinsurance.com/article/20120819/NEWS06/308199985.

Tuana, Nancy. 2004. "Coming to Understand: Orgasm and the Epistemology of Ignorance." *Hypatia* 19 (1): 194–232. doi:10.1111/j.1527-2001.2004.tb01275.x.

———. 2006. "The Speculum of Ignorance: The Women's Health Movement and Epistemologies of Ignorance." *Hypatia* 21 (3): 1–19. doi:10.1111/j.1527-2001.2006.tb01110.x.

Uhlenberg, Peter. 2013. "Demography Is Not Destiny: The Challenges and Opportunities of Global Population Aging." *Generations* 37 (1): 12–19.

Uitto, Juha. 1998. "The Geography in Megacities: A Theoretical Framework." *Applied Geography* 18 (I): 7–16.

Uitto, Juha, and Rajib Shaw. 2006. "Adaptation to Changing Climate: Promoting Community-Based Approaches in the Developing Countries." *Sansai* 1:93–108.

UNFCC. 2015. "Historic Paris Agreement on Climate Change." http://newsroom.unfccc.int/unfccc-newsroom/finale-cop21/.

"United Nations Climate Change Conference Paris 2015." 2015. http://www.un.org/sustainabledevelopment/cop21/.

"U.S. Army Corps of Engineers Jacksonville District JUNE 2010." 2010. Vol. I. Jacksonville.

"US Census Quick Facts Puerto Rico." 2016. US Census. https://www.census.gov/quickfacts/fact/table/PR/AGE775216#viewtop.

"The U.S. Population Living at the Coast." 2012. National Oceanic and Atmospheric Administration. http://stateofthecoast.noaa.gov/population/welcome.html.

Valle-Levinson, Arnoldo, Andrea Dutton, and Jonathan B. Martin. 2017. "Spatial and Temporal Variability of Sea Level Rise Hot Spots over the Eastern United States." *Geophysical Research Letters* 44 (15): 7876–82. doi:10.1002/2017GL073926.

Van Someren, Eus J. W. 2007. "Thermoregulation and Aging." *American Journal of Physiology: Regulatory, Integrative and Comparative Physiology* 292 (1): R99–102. doi:10.1152/ajpregu.00557.2006.

Venciana-Suarez, Ana. 2017. "Walk of Death? Florida Is the Most Dangerous Place for Pedestrians." *Miami Herald*, January 10. http://www.miamiherald.com/news/local/article12558 8259.html.

Vincent, G. K., and V. A Velkoff. 2010. "The Next Four Decades: The Older Population in the United States: 2010 to 2050." Washington, DC: U.S. Census Bureau. https://www.census.gov/library/publications/2010/demo/p25-1138.html.

Wadhams, Peter. 2013. "Diminishing Sea-Ice Extent and Thickness in the Arctic Ocean." In *Environmental Security in the Arctic Ocean*, edited by P. A. Vylegzhanin and A. N. Berkman, 15–30. Dordrecht: Springer Link. doi:10.1007/978-94-007-4713-5_4.

Wall Street Journal. 2009. "Tax My Products, Please." March 17. http://online.wsj.com/news/articles/SB123725594071950875.

Wang, Amy, Cleve R. Wootson, and Ed O'Keefe. 2017. "As Harvey Submerges Houston, Local Officials Defend Their Calls Not to Evacuate." *Washington Post*, August 28. https://www.washingtonpost.com/news/post-nation/wp/2017/08/27/harvey-is-causing-epic-catastrophic-flooding-in-houston-why-wasnt-the-city-evacuated/?utm_term=.458f177e 5866.

Wang, Chunzai, and Sang-Ki Lee. 2008. "Global Warming and United States Landfalling Hurricanes." *Geophysical Research Letters* 35 (2): L02708. doi:10.1029/2007GL032396.

Washington, Wayne, Corvaya Jefferies, Andrew Marra, and Joe Capozzi. 2017. "Hurricane Irma: Employees Question County Shelter Staffing Policy." *Palm Beach Post*, September 15. http://www.mypalmbeachpost.com/weather/hurricanes/hurricane-irma-employees-question-county-shelter-staffing-policy/wG98W3kYnvgS3jSwW76QBN/.

Watson-Jones, Rachel, and Cristine Legare. 2016. "The Social Functions of Group Rituals." *Current Directions in Psychological Science* 25 (1): 42–46. doi: 10.1177/096372141 5618486.

Wdowinski, Shimon, Ronald Bray, Ben P. Kirtman, and Zhaohua Wu. 2016. "Increasing Flooding Hazard in Coastal Communities Due to Rising Sea Level: Case Study of Miami Beach, Florida." *Ocean & Coastal Management* 126 (June): 1–8. doi:10.1016/j.ocecoa man.2016.03.002.

Webb, Brian S., and Doug Hayhoe. 2017. "Assessing the Influence of an Educational Presentation on Climate Change Beliefs at an Evangelical Christian College." *Journal of Geoscience Education* 65 (3): 272–82. doi:10.5408/16-220.1.

Wells, Ken. 2008. *The Good Pirates of the Forgotten Bayous: Fighting to Save a Way of Life in the Wake of Hurricane Katrina*. New Haven, CT: Yale University Press.

White, Nancy M., and Richard A. Weinstein. 2008. "The Mexican Connection and the Far West of the U.S. Southeast." *American Antiquity* 72 (2): 227.

Whitehouse, Peter J., Atwood D. Gaines, Heather Lindstrom, and Janice E. Graham. 2005. "Anthropological Contributions to the Understanding of Age-Related Cognitive Impairment." *Lancet Neurology* 4 (5): 320–26. http://www.thelancet.com/journals/laneur/article/PIIS1474-4422(05)70075-2/abstract.

Wiist, William. 2011. "Citizens United, Public Health, and Democracy: The Supreme Court Ruling, Its Implications, and Proposed Action." *American Journal of Public Health* 101 (7): 1172–79. doi:10.2105/AJPH.2010.300043.

Williams, Perry. 2017. "Australia's Turnbull Wins Promise of More Gas from Energy Majors." *Bloomberg News*, March 15. https://www.bloomberg.com/news/articles/2017-03-15/australia-s-turnbull-wins-promise-of-more-gas-from-energy-majors-j0bnwhj6.

Wisner, Ben, Piers Blaikie, Terry Cannon, and Ian Davis. 2004. *At Risk: Natural Hazards, People's Vulnerability and Disasters*, 2nd ed. New York: Routledge.

Wisner, Ben, and Juha Uitto. 2009. "Life on the Edge: Urban Social Vulnerability and Decentralized, Citizen-Based Disaster Risk Reduction in Four Large Cities of the Pacific Rim." In *Facing Global Environmental Change*, edited by H. G. Brauch, N. C. Behera, P. Kameri-Mbote, J. Grin, U. Oswald Spring, B. Chourou, C. Mesjasz, and H. Krummenacher, 215–31. AFES Press.

"WMO Provisional Statement on the State of Global Climate in 2017." 2017, 4–5. http://ane4bf-datap1.s3-eu-west-1.amazonaws.com/wmocms/s3fs-public/ckeditor/files/2017_provisional_statement_text_-_updated_04Nov2017_1.pdf?7rBjqhMTRJkQbvuYMNAmetvBgFeyS_vQ.

Womack, Mari. 2010. *The Anthropology of Health and Healing*. Lanham, MD: Altamira Press.

Woodruff, Jonathan D., Jennifer L. Irish, and Suzana J. Camargo. 2013. "Coastal Flooding by Tropical Cyclones and Sea-Level Rise." *Nature* 504 (7478): 44–52. doi:10.1038/nature12855.

Wright, Daniel B., Thomas R. Knutson, and James A. Smith. 2015. "Regional Climate Model Projections of Rainfall from U.S. Landfalling Tropical Cyclones." *Climate Dynamics* 45 (11–12): 3365–79. doi:10.1007/s00382-015-2544-y.

Xu, X., X. Zuo, X. Wang, and S. Han. 2009. "Do You Feel My Pain? Racial Group Membership Modulates Empathic Neural Responses." *Journal of Neuroscience* 29 (26): 8525–29. doi:10.1523/JNEUROSCI.2418-09.2009.

Yen, Irene H., and Lynda A. Anderson. 2012. "Built Environment and Mobility of Older Adults: Important Policy and Practice Efforts." *Journal of the American Geriatrics Society* 60 (5): 951–56. doi:10.1111/j.1532-5415.2012.03949.x.

Zanona, Melanie. 2017. "White House Lets Jones Act Waiver Expire for Puerto Rico." *The Hill*, October 9. http://thehill.com/latino/354561-white-house-lets-jones-act-waiver-expire-for-puerto-rico.

Zhang, K., C. Xiao, and S. P. Leatherman. 2006. "Storm Surge Simulation for Lake Okeechobee. Report to Florida Department of Community Affairs."

Index

About the Author

Janelle Christensen's research interests lie at the intersection of disaster management and aging studies, exploring how community dwelling families respond to emergency preparedness and disaster planning while simultaneously providing care for family members with Alzheimer's disease. She completed both a PhD in applied biocultural anthropology and a master's in public health (MPH) at the University of South Florida. She also has an MA in sociology of law from the International Institute for Sociology of Law in Oñati, Spain. Her sociolegal research was conducted in intentional communities (Camphill Communities) based on the care of individuals with developmental disabilities in Germany and the United States. Christensen works in the Institutional Research division at Florida Southwestern State College, where she teaches anthropology and sociology courses. She is also an independent contractor, assisting with data analysis for gerontological health projects.

www.ingramcontent.com/pod-product-compliance
Lightning Source LLC
Chambersburg PA
CBHW020001290326
41935CB00007B/264